HAPPY GUT

HAPPY GUT

THE CLEANSING PROGRAM
TO HELP YOU LOSE WEIGHT,
GAIN ENERGY, AND ELIMINATE PAIN

Dr. Vincent Pedre

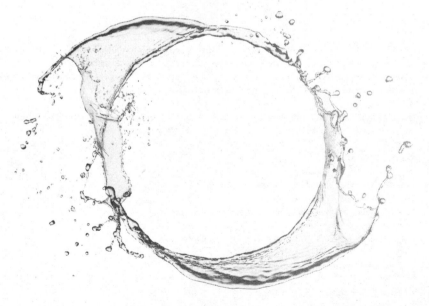

wm
WILLIAM MORROW
An Imprint of HarperCollins*Publishers*

HarperCollins books may be purchased for educational, business, or sales promotional use. For information please e-mail the Special Markets Department at SPsales@harpercollins.com.

FIRST EDITION

Title page photograph © by Thomas Vogel / Getty Images

Part title pages Waves provided by StudioSmart/Shutterstock, Inc.

Diagrams on pages 17, 22, 23, 98, and 122 © by Ryan Gibboney 2015

Photographs in Chapter 8 by Joseph Rettberg

Designed by Lisa Stokes

Library of Congress Cataloging-in-Publication Data has been applied for.

ISBN 978-0-06-236216-2

15 16 17 18 19 ov/rrd 10 9 8 7 6 5 4 3 2 1

To my mother—I know you would be so proud.

To my father—Thank you for giving me the opportunity to become a doctor and help others.

And to my son, Ambrose—May you always have a happy gut.

CONTENTS

FOREWORD
Leo Galland, MD

Author of *The Allergy Solution: The Surprising, Hidden Truth About Why You Are Sick and How to Get Well*

NEW YORK, NEW YORK

THE MAIN THING YOU want from your digestive tract is that it does its job quietly, without talking back to you. You don't want to know that it's there.

As Dr. Vincent Pedre explains in *Happy Gut*, that job is actually much bigger than you've ever imagined. Not only is the gastrointestinal system responsible for digesting and absorbing nutrients from food and for excreting waste, it is also the largest organ of your immune system. Over two-thirds of your body's lymphocytes (the captains of immune function) are found in the lining of the small intestine. From this base they travel throughout your body, sending signals that influence immunity in all other organs.

Your gastrointestinal tract has its own nervous system, technically called the Enteric Nervous System (ENS) and affectionately dubbed "The Second Brain" by aficionados. Your ENS has as many nerve cells as your spinal cord and is in constant communication with your first brain, affecting your mood and mental function.

Your alimentary canal is also home to about a hundred trillion microbes, which include a thousand different species of bacteria, a few dozen types of yeasts and fungi, an unknown number of viruses, and an occasional worm. Collectively these are called the "gut microbiome." Understanding how these microbes influence human health and illness has been a major interest of mine for over three decades. In the last decade, microbiome research has blossomed into one of the most-discussed topics in applied science. It's become clear that gut microbes help us to be human. The implications of that relationship will be at the cutting edge of clinical research for decades to come.

Finally, the gastrointestinal tract is an organ of detoxification. Much of this responsibility rests with the liver, but the intestinal lining cells themselves are rich in detoxifying enzymes. The gut and liver work together to remove noxious substances derived from food, your environment, gut microbes, and even the operation of your own metabolism and hormones.

These multiple functions of the digestive system interact with each other and with the food you eat to regulate your nutritional state, your metabolic state, your mental state, your weight, your pattern of sleep, your energy, and your susceptibility to illness. *Happy Gut* is an engaging guide to your most complex organ system, the GI tract, and a gold mine of practical information that allows you to help this system work for you, instead of against you.

Dr. Pedre pays special attention to the practical details that allow you to apply his Gut C.A.R.E. Program effectively. If you're following his advice and wonder, "How do I go about doing this?", you'll find that he's anticipated your question and provided the answer. Just keep reading.

Another outstanding feature of *Happy Gut* is the attention it pays to important topics that don't receive enough consideration in most self-help books for digestive disorders. These include:

• **The Gut-Brain Connection.** Dr. Pedre explains how gut microbes and gut toxins influence your brain and how your mind affects the function of your gut. The detailed descriptions of mindful eating and yoga for G.I. health are wonderful.

• **The benefits of stomach acid.** He emphasizes the importance of stomach acid for normal digestion and describes the many dangers of acid-suppressing drugs, the third largest-selling drug category in the world.

• **Prebiotics.** Prebiotics are food components that are not digested or absorbed in your GI tract. They travel through your gut supporting the growth of beneficial bacteria. Many people take prebiotic powders as dietary supplements. Dr. Pedre tells you how you can get them from food.

• **Laboratory testing.** Throughout *Happy Gut*, you'll find detailed information about laboratory testing that can help you and your doctor identify factors that are creating your symptoms. This knowledge can help you partner more effectively with your personal health care provider.

• **Food sensitivity.** Dr. Pedre starts with a thoughtful discussion of specific foods that should be avoided and why. He then shows you how to listen to the wisdom of your body as you reintroduce foods you've removed. Understanding the difference between food sensitivity and food allergy is essential for discovering your optimal diet, which may be different from someone else's optimal diet.

If you want to improve your digestive health, you should read every word in this book.

INTRODUCTION

The gut is your own internal garden.

—DR. MARK HYMAN

*T*WENTY-SIX-YEAR-OLD *Julie has tried all types of diets and seen several doctors (including two gastroenterologists), but no one has offered a true solution to her symptoms. She suffers on a daily basis from gas, bloating, indigestion, and irregular or urgent bowels, sometimes having to run to the bathroom in the middle of a dinner out with friends, which causes her great embarrassment. She says that because of her unpredictable stomach, "it feels like food just goes right through me." She is bloated and holding on to ten pounds she cannot easily shed.*

Her discomfort began several years before we met, while she was attending college. She admits to having had "not the best diet" during her college years, and she frequently snacked on chips, pizza, beer, and late-night sweets while studying. There was no clear start date for her symptoms, but they slowly got worse over the years, and now Julie is at the point that she cannot get a handle on what upsets her stomach and when. She is afraid to go out because of it, and this has really put a damper on her social life. She will stay home on most weekend nights because she simply cannot predict how she will feel.

She had blood work and even a colonoscopy (a procedure where a specialist looks into the colon with a long, tubelike camera), but no test has revealed why she feels this way. When she came to see me, she was at her wits' end, in tears, and wondering if she would ever feel normal again.

You may be reading Julie's story and thinking, "This sounds like me." Or perhaps you relate to some of her symptoms. You may have visited multiple doctors while seeking an answer to your complaints, only to find disappointment—being sent home either empty-handed or with a prescription for your symptoms or an antidepressant, but not with a diagnosis of the cause. "It's all in my head," you think, because the doctor told you there was no identifiable physical ailment. To complicate matters more, in many cases these symptoms (gas, bloating, alternating constipation/diarrhea, and abdominal discomfort relieved by bowel movements) get placed under the umbrella term "Irritable Bowel Syndrome" (IBS), which gives them a name but does nothing to clarify the true cause or the treatment. This happened to Julie and may have happened to you. Many gut issues suffer the same consequences.

The doctor may say, "Your colon looks perfectly normal. It's probably just stress. Diet has nothing to do with it. Go home, try to relax, and your symptoms will improve over time." The truth is, many doctors simply don't know what tests to order, and they know much less about nutrition and how diet may be a major culprit in your symptoms.

I used to be one of those nutritionally challenged medical doctors. When I went to medical school, nutrition was a brief side note to the more "important" time spent learning how drugs treat disease. (Lucky for all of us, that is now changing in medical schools.)

Of course, I knew nutritional macro-concepts, like eating hormone-free meats and organic fruits and vegetables was cleaner and healthier, but I didn't realize how damaging dietary indiscretions could be, or how what is right for one person may be wrong for another person.

My story began long before medical school, when I was a child. I had a "nervous stomach." Whenever I had a test or a piano performance, I had a swarm of "butterflies" doing somersaults inside my belly. I would feel so sick to my stomach that I had to eat long before any stressful events or I might risk vomiting. I suffered from "weak digestion" and caught upper respiratory infections that turned into bronchitis so frequently that my pediatrician was concerned about my immune system and prescribed a multivitamin, thinking that it would strengthen my defenses. Little did my parents (nor my doctor, for that matter) know that the milk, sugar-laden wheat cereals, and milkshakes they were feeding me (after all, milk makes for strong bones and helps you grow) were hurting my stomach and weakening my immune system. It wasn't until I was in my early twenties, when I stopped having cereal with milk for breakfast simply because it was not convenient for my busy student lifestyle, that I ceased getting sick as regularly. All those years I had believed, like most of us do, that milk was good for me. It was eye-opening to realize that this was not the case, and it was more than just lactose intolerance.

By then I was in medical school, and I started making the connection that diet played a stronger role in how I felt than I realized. It was hard to believe that my friends could eat the same foods as I did but have none of the secondary effects I was feeling. With a few changes, including adding more healthy fats to my diet, I felt better than I ever had before, but as much as I had improved, I still wasn't in the clear. It took several more years to fully grasp the best way to eat for my body.

What began as a nervous stomach in my childhood turned into IBS by my mid-to-late twenties. I'd learned to control my nerves through meditation, but stress often led to frequent, soft stools. Yes, I know, gross! But we have to talk about poop, because therein lay the problem.

I was not getting sick as often with upper respiratory infections, but I was still eating some of the wrong foods (I was as much subject to the powerful marketing of the food industry in the United States as we all are). I was eating all the foods that are part of the accepted Western diet. These included meats, fruits, vegetables, and salads, but also pizza, bread, bagels, sandwiches, and pasta. I had no idea that gluten was my enemy. Without symptoms I was aware of, how could I?

Eating wheat is so ingrained in our culture that while I was in my residency training at Mount Sinai Hospital in New York City, the sponsored lunch meal for our noontime lectures was often . . . guess what? Pizza and soda! Talk about a power combo that would certainly put us into a food coma! When you're on a food and time budget, these foods are the cheapest and quickest, and when you're stressed and studying or working into the late-night or early-morning hours, they are the types of foods that are not only tasty but also comforting to eat. In fact, sleep-deprivation studies have shown that participants begin craving starchy, sugary foods the longer they stay awake. If we were lucky, a salad option was available once in a while. Again, seeing this way of eating as the norm made it harder for me to realize how damaging it was. Little did I know that my diet was contributing to inflammation and a leaky gut. I was exhausted, but I didn't know why.

As I started experimenting with dietary changes to improve how I felt, I realized that I felt my best when eating lean, organic meats and lots of fresh vegetables. I experimented by getting rid of all processed foods from my diet, buying only organic, and cooking most of my meals at home. Within two weeks, the improvement in my energy levels and general sense of well-being was striking! I knew I was onto something, but as good as those changes were, they still were not enough. To truly conquer my gut symptoms I had to heal my leaky gut. And conquering your unhappy gut is what I want to help you do as well with *Happy Gut*.

So where do we begin? Let's start by looking at why your gut is so unhappy. This book is meant to break through the veil of frustration that so often surrounds these unanswered symptoms.

Part I covers how you got here; in other words, how your gut was thrown out of balance, what these imbalances cause, and which foods are the most troublesome and why.

- Chapter 1 looks at how your gut became so imbalanced and how the Gut C.A.R.E. Program can help you fix that in twenty-eight days. You will see how gut health is connected to weight gain and how eliminating the top food allergens or food sensitivities in the Happy Gut Diet translates into easy, seamless weight loss without counting calories. I also explain why the Western model fails us and present a new paradigm for explaining gut symptoms. This paradigm, the Functional Medicine approach, is embodied in the Gut C.A.R.E. Program.

- Chapter 2 shows you what foods are in or out in the Happy Gut Diet. You'll learn why you need to avoid certain foods—foods that you probably eat every day and that are making you feel tired and swollen without your realizing it, causing you to gain weight or plateau in your weight-loss efforts.

In Part II, we'll begin to heal your gut with our gut "reboot" system: the Gut C.A.R.E. Program.

- Chapter 3 will give you an overview of the Happy Gut Diet and teach you my step-by-step plan—the Gut C.A.R.E. Program—for fixing your unruly gut and gut-associated conditions for good.

- Chapter 4 gives you my top tips for success while on the program, including a list of common questions and answers.

In Part III, we explore the post–Happy Gut Diet food Reintroduction Phase as well as further tests that can help clarify your underlying issues.

- In Chapter 5, we look at how to phase back into a normal diet after the twenty-eight-day Happy Gut Diet. I also give you the tools and strategies to manage your gut with an individualized and doable lifelong plan.

- Chapter 6 looks at the underlying causes and symptoms for many common and some not-so-common gut ailments. It is a guide for looking deeper into your gut-related issues after you are done with the Gut C.A.R.E. Program.

In Part IV, we look at the emotional and physical connections to gut health, including how an unhealthy gut can lead to many psychological disorders, including depression, attention deficit disorder, and autism. To achieve true wellness, there must be an alignment of the mind, body, and spirit, and I share simple, effective strategies that have worked for my patients.

- Chapter 7 discusses the mind-gut connection and how the gut really does act as our "second brain." This important information can be used in how we approach common conditions, such as depression. We'll also explore alternative modalities—including acupuncture, reflexology, Reiki, and massage, to name a few—that can serve as an important part of an integrative approach to healing and maintaining a healthy gut.

- In Chapter 8, you'll learn how movement and meditation benefit long-term gut healing and health. I share seven daily yoga poses for gut health from my yoga teachers and gurus, Paula Tursi and Janet Dailey Butler, along with positive affirmations and breath work to help you balance and reduce your stress response.

In Part V, we head to the Happy Gut Kitchen.

- Chapter 9 offers tasty, gut-friendly recipes developed with chef Mikaela Reuben and chef/dietician Marlisa Brown to get you on the way to living with a *happy gut*. These delicious recipes will show you how easy it is to prepare *Happy Gut*–approved meals while still avoiding the high-sensitivity foods that were wreaking havoc in your body.

- I conclude *Happy Gut* with helpful tools and resources. The Appendices include tools to assist you in getting through the program, including food and symptom journals, a health timeline, a post-program questionnaire, recommended supplements, and a list of important resources you will want to check out to continue this journey.

Many of my patients come to see me after they have been suffering from gut-associated symptoms for years. Others are looking for ways to lose weight while becoming healthier. With the Gut C.A.R.E. Program, the Happy Gut Diet, patience, and understanding, you can conquer your gut symptoms and gut-associated maladies for good, helping you to alter the course of a chronic disease, lose weight, gain energy, and eliminate abdominal and generalized body aches and pain!

Are you ready? Let's improve your health and get you on the path to a *happy gut*!

IT'S ALL ABOUT THE GUT

IT'S ALL IN YOUR GUT

At the heart of every order and disorder is inflammation.

—DR. DAVID PERLMUTTER

YOU WAKE UP IN the morning and your gut is bloated from the night before. You haven't had a bowel movement in days, and you're praying that today will be the day—and soon, before you go to work. Your worst nightmare is a sudden need to rush to the bathroom while on your way to the office, when you'll have to find a decent public restroom. You're exhausted, your joints hurt, your body aches, and your muscles are tender. You have your third headache or migraine this month. Your ability to concentrate seems like a skill from your distant past. Your days are controlled by stimulants (caffeine) and relaxants (the foods you're addicted to or a beer or glass of wine every night)— each morning you wake up feeling no better, but you repeat the cycle because you think it's the only way you can make it through the day. What you might not know is that at the root of your malaise is a gut out of balance.

WHAT MAKES A HEALTHY GUT

Your gut is your internal garden and requires tending just like a garden would. As your skin forms a barrier to the world *outside* your body, your gut plays a similar role *inside* your body. Its surface area is a remarkable

200 times greater than that of your skin, making it your largest surface of interaction with the outside world. The gut is in continuous contact with nutrients, as well as all types of toxins, food additives, microbes, and drugs that may pass through your digestive tract on a daily basis. As gatekeeper, your gut has a huge task to not only serve as a porous filter for the building blocks of life, but also to keep out all the detrimental substances you may be exposed to.

Within the healthy gut lives a world of friendly bacteria that help us digest, produce vitamins, stimulate a vibrant gut lining, and keep unfriendly organisms in check. Signals from the gut to the brain tell you when you are full so that you do not overeat. You feel satiated but not overfull after meals. Digestion moves from the mouth to the rectum in a well-orchestrated series of steps. Just the right amount of digestive juices are secreted and at the right time. And bowel movements occur at least once daily so that waste and toxins are efficiently removed from the body via the stool.

A healthy gut is one where:

- All food is digested into its component parts
- The digestive surface is vibrant and able to absorb micronutrients while blocking the entrance of larger, partially digested food particles; bacteria; yeast; and parasites
- The gut-associated immune system is activated only when necessary and is not overstimulated

DIGESTION 101

Digestion begins in the mouth when you start chewing your food. Saliva starts to break down the carbohydrates in the food. The food then travels down your esophagus into the stomach. The low pH (high acid) environment in the stomach activates peptidases (enzymes) that begin to break down any protein. The acid environment is also a first line of defense against bacteria, parasites, and yeast that you may inadvertently ingest. Peptidases work best in an acid environment. Carbohydrates break down into glucose. Protein is broken down into amino acids—the building blocks of muscle and tissue. Then, as the food moves into the small intestine, the pH changes from acid to more alkaline as bile is secreted from the liver/gallbladder to emulsify fats for absorption. The process continues throughout the length of the small intestine, where bacteria that naturally live in our gut begin fermenting and feeding off the food we eat. They help us break it down, sometimes in unfavorable ways that produce lots of gas, but also in ways that help us, like producing necessary vitamins. The food then travels to the colon, where water is absorbed from the digested food/bacterial mass, producing the final product: a well-formed stool. Many things can go wrong in this process, and that is what we are going to explore in later chapters.

PRIMARY ORGANS OF DIGESTION

- **Liver:** Produces bile, which serves to emulsify and absorb fats. It is also the primary organ of detoxification, processing all toxins absorbed from the environment as well as drugs and our own hormones.
- **Gallbladder:** Stores bile and secretes a small amount into the small intestine during a meal.
- **Pancreas:** Secretes pancreatic juice, which is alkaline, to neutralize the acid from the stomach. Mainly contains lipases and proteases, which help break down proteins and fat. The pancreas also produces important hormones, like insulin, that are involved in the regulation of nutrients in the bloodstream.

The Five Key Roles of the Gut

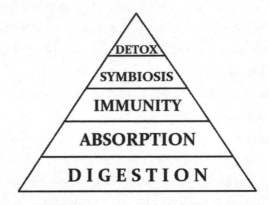

Your gut has five key roles:

1. **Digestion** of food
2. **Absorption** of nutrients
3. Maintenance of an **immune barrier** to the outside world
4. A **symbiotic** relationship with favorable bacteria
5. **Detoxification,** which includes the elimination of waste and toxins from the body

The moment each of us passed through the birth canal, a unique combination of microbes from our mother's vagina initiated the process of colonizing our bodies, both inside in our airways and digestive tract and outside on our skin.[1] Thus began the long process of bacterial colonization, first with our mother's bacteria, and then continuing throughout our lives by our exposures to the environment. Our bacterial colonies change depending on our lifestyle, what we eat, and our exposures to antibiotics. The state of this internal microbial milieu literally dictates how our bodies feel, how our immune systems behave, and how we digest and assimilate foods.

FACTS ABOUT THE GUT MICROBIOME

- There are ten times as many microbial cells in our bodies as our own cells.
- The gut microbiome contains up to 150 times as many genes as the genetic pool inside human cells.

Unfortunately the dietary contribution of the Standard American Diet (SAD), which is full of sugar, processed foods, and food additives, promotes the growth of harmful bacteria and yeast. It also turns on genes that are unfavorable for your well-being. When I say it all starts in your gut, I mean almost everything! Headaches, migraines, allergies, autoimmunity, weight gain, acne, skin rashes, yeast infections, hormonal imbalances, fatigue, immune challenges, even the way you sense pain—they all relate to the condition and health of your gut.

FUNCTIONAL MEDICINE VS. WESTERN MEDICINE

Functional medicine is about creating *resiliency* in the human body.
—*Dr. Mark Hyman, speech at the Institute for
Functional Medicine's 2014 Annual International Conference*

Now that we've made the connection between your gut and the rest of your symptoms, let's look at how the Functional Medicine model and the Gut C.A.R.E. Program provide a powerful and thorough alternative, often more successful than the Western approach, to heal gut-related issues.

A drawback in Western medicine is that it often treats symptoms but not their causes. It gives a disease or combination of symptoms a name (like "IBS"), but that doesn't bring the doctor or the patient closer to the root causes of the problem. The name fails to explain the underlying imbalances that led to the symptoms in the first place.

Whereas Western medicine is symptom and diagnosis centered, Functional Medicine is patient and process centered. Western medicine strives to eliminate symptoms, whereas Functional Medicine endeavors to enhance and support the innate ability of the body to heal itself. It treats the individual as a system—like a symphony orchestra. Any underlying imbalance in one part will be felt throughout the entire system, the same way an out-of-tune or out-of-sync instrument will set an entire orchestra off. With Functional Medicine, the focus is on identifying and addressing the underlying causes of the problem and bringing them back into harmony. That is done, in part, by understanding how systems (your body) function and how to address them when they malfunction.

THE PROBLEM WITH ACID BLOCKERS

A case in point in the Western versus Functional Medicine approach is proton pump inhibitors (PPIs)—a class of drugs used to treat acid reflux, ulcers, and gastritis. If you take these drugs long term, they may lead to calcium malabsorption, osteoporosis, bone fractures, and B_{12} deficiency, among other secondary effects.

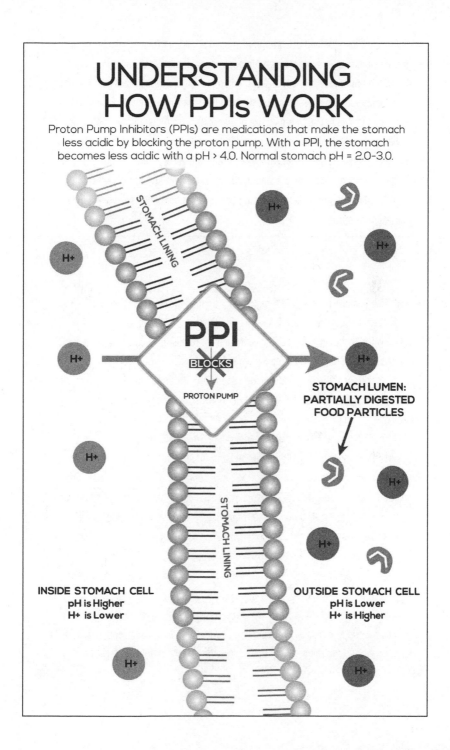

UNDERSTANDING HOW PPIs WORK

Proton Pump Inhibitors (PPIs) are medications that make the stomach less acidic by blocking the proton pump. With a PPI, the stomach becomes less acidic with a pH > 4.0. Normal stomach pH = 2.0-3.0.

STOMACH LINING

H+

PPI
X
BLOCKS
PROTON PUMP

STOMACH LUMEN:
PARTIALLY DIGESTED
FOOD PARTICLES

STOMACH LINING

INSIDE STOMACH CELL
pH is Higher
H+ is Lower

OUTSIDE STOMACH CELL
pH is Lower
H+ is Higher

Raising the stomach pH with an acid blocker (like a PPI or H$_2$ blocker, which includes medications like Nexium, Prilosec, Zantac, and Cimetidine) not only hinders proper digestion, but it also creates fertile ground for yeast (like *Candida*) to colonize your digestive tract, particularly the small intestine. These unfriendly yeast can be the cause of a plethora of symptoms, from chronic fatigue to muscle aches, joint pains, mental fog, abdominal discomfort and bloating, anal itching, and skin rashes. Often these symptoms are treated in Western medicine as just that—symptoms. But they are merely the tip of the iceberg. What's underlying is an imbalanced gut, which is causing you to feel a combination of seemingly unrelated symptoms.

We often confuse treating the symptoms for treating the disease. If you had a leaky faucet, would you reach for a bucket to "fix" the leak, or look for the root cause—a loose valve—and tighten it to resolve the leak? Frequently, Western doctors are reaching for the bucket without looking under the sink.

In contrast, Functional Medicine recognizes the mechanisms through which things happen in the body, allowing us to work at the core level to heal the body.

A perfect example of this is the story of my patient Katherine.

When thirty-two-year-old Katherine came to see me, she was suffering from multiple loose, sometimes bloody stools daily and lots of abdominal pain no matter what she ate, and she was feeling down and depressed. She could not get a handle on her symptoms and thought they were stress induced. I knew something was going on in her colon with the history of blood in her stools, but I suspected there was more to it than that. I drew labs to rule out other underlying causes and found that she had positive markers for celiac disease (a type of severe autoimmune gluten intolerance). I sent her to my colleague, a GI specialist, who performed both an endoscopy and a colonoscopy. Through the biopsies, we found that she had ulcerative colitis, a form of inflammatory bowel disease, and confirmed the diagnosis of celiac disease. I had already put her on an anti-

inflammatory, gluten-free diet and the Gut C.A.R.E. Program, including working on reducing her stress and encouraging her to learn to cook at home. She began to improve. It took several months to help her fully recover, but with diligence she was able to regain her gut health.

In this case, both Western medicine and Functional Medicine worked cooperatively to help Katherine mend in the quickest and best way possible. This is the ideal way that Functional Medicine and Western medicine should be used—not in opposition to each other, but cooperatively to provide the best possible state-of-the-art care.[2]

FOOD IS INFORMATION

If you want to get to the root causes of what is going on inside your gut, you need to look at what you're putting at the end of your fork. Food is information. From the biochemical reactions that occur at the cellular level to what you see and feel in your body as a whole, the types of foods you eat can actually turn on or off good or bad genes. If you consume a milkshake, hamburger, and French fries, you will turn on genes that promote inflammation in your gut and your body, whereas if you eat two cups of steamed broccoli, you will turn on anticancer and anti-inflammatory gene pathways.

The foods we eat control our state of health, and the gut is the gateway to the rest of the body. Who's ultimately in control of that gateway? Let me give you a hint. Look in the mirror. You are—by what you put in your mouth. Well, that's only part of the truth.

The Addictive Nature of Processed Foods

Your food choices aren't all under your control. There is an addictive nature to some foods that can take control of your cravings. We've become accustomed to eating foods that are far removed from where they grew, as well as foods that are processed and overprocessed. School programs that help educate children about where their food comes from, even teaching them how to grow their own vegetable gardens, have proven that knowing the source of their food increases the likelihood that children will make healthy choices when eating.

However, the food industry looks to sabotage our healthier inclinations. It has preyed on brain chemistry by researching and designing the combinations of salty, sweet, and fat that make food so addictive that it's tremendously difficult to stop at one or two bites. It has also made it hard to understand what is inside our food by using deceptive labeling.

The same principles are used by large restaurant chains to make their food more pleasing and addictive. If you have never watched the documentary *Super Size Me,* I highly recommend that you do. I think you will be shocked to see how these foods cause damage to our internal organs (like the liver), while at the same time making our brains crave even more.

One of the most common cravings is sugar. For this reason, you may eat too much sugar without realizing it. Perhaps you love to eat carbohydrates (like bread, rice, and pasta), which basically turn into sugar as a result of digestion. You may like to drink fruit and vegetable juices because you think they're good for you—without realizing how much fruit sugar you are consuming. You are unknowingly feeding yeast and unfriendly bacteria in your gut, then wondering why you don't feel well.

The only way to break the cycle is to stop eating these foods. *Happy Gut* will help you do that. Not only will you learn to stop eating the foods that are upsetting your digestive system and causing weight gain, pain, and fatigue, but you will also overcome your desire and cravings for the foods that are slowly making you sick.

OTHER REASONS YOUR GUT IS UNHAPPY

Your gut is also unhappy because of stress. Research shows the stress response can alter the natural balance of healthy bacteria in your gut, causing the gut ecology to shift in favor of a more hostile group of bacteria. When patients with gut issues come in to see me, I ask what they do to relieve and manage their stress, and often they say, "Nothing." Many people lack this level of self-care. They believe they don't have the time, but as I'll explain in Chapters 7 and 8, incorporating meditation and yoga as part of a daily routine can take as little as ten minutes, and those few minutes will pay off with big rewards for your gut and general sense of well-being.

Then there is the problem of antibiotics. Antibiotics are simply over-prescribed. As a physician, I can tell you that the majority of infections that are seen by primary doctors are viral. Most antibiotics only kill bacteria. Except for a select few, viruses are unaffected by antibiotics. Most colds (including early sinus infections and bronchitis) are caused by viruses and will resolve on their own without antibiotic therapy, yet people continuously request antibiotics within the first two days of the onset of cold symptoms to "knock it out." Most of the time, rest and immune support are enough to resolve these infections. Knowing the damage that antibiotics inflict on our gut flora, I struggle to get my patients to understand that not all infections require antibiotics. The big picture is that the overuse of antibiotics is leading to more antibiotic-resistant bugs that are difficult to treat and can claim lives.

That said, most everyone has been on multiple courses of antibiotics throughout his or her lifetime. Each time you take antibiotics, your gut flora is altered. Then, if you don't eat the right foods, including cultured or fermented foods, you inevitably suffer from a dysbiosis—an imbalance between favorable and unfavorable microorganisms in the gut.

HOW DYSBIOSIS LEADS TO ILLNESS

Dysbiosis is a microbial imbalance generally inside the gut, characterized by increased levels of harmful bacteria, yeast and/or parasites, and reduced levels of beneficial bacteria.

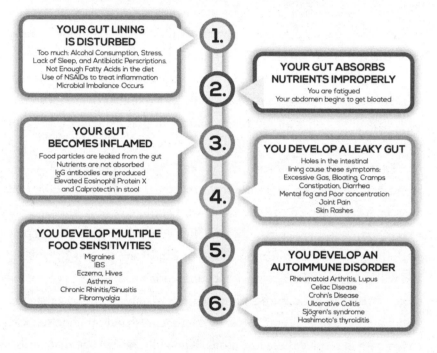

1.

YOUR GUT LINING IS DISTURBED

Too much: Alcohol Consumption, Stress, Lack of Sleep, and Antibiotic Perscriptions.
Not Enough Fatty Acids in the diet
Use of NSAIDs to treat inflammation
Microbial Imbalance Occurs

2.

YOUR GUT ABSORBS NUTRIENTS IMPROPERLY

You are fatigued
Your abdomen begins to get bloated

3.

YOUR GUT BECOMES INFLAMED

Food particles are leaked from the gut
Nutrients are not absorbed
IgG antibodies are produced
Elevated Eosinophil Protein X
and Calprotectin in stool

YOU DEVELOP A LEAKY GUT

Holes in the intestinal
lining cause these symptoms:
Excessive Gas, Bloating, Cramps
Constipation, Diarrhea
Mental fog and Poor concentration
Joint Pain
Skin Rashes

4.

YOU DEVELOP MULTIPLE FOOD SENSITIVITIES

Migraines
IBS
Eczema, Hives
Asthma
Chronic Rhinitis/Sinusitis
Fibromyalgia

5.

YOU DEVELOP AN AUTOIMMUNE DISORDER

Rheumatoid Arthritis, Lupus
Celiac Disease
Crohn's Disease
Ulcerative Colitis
Sjögren's syndrome
Hashimoto's thyroiditis

6.

Between the antibiotics, eating the wrong foods that feed the bad organisms, the toxins you are exposed to in your environment, and the resulting dysbiosis, over a period of days to months you develop a leaky gut. This leakiness or "hyperpermeability" exposes your body to partially digested protein molecules from food. The immune system does not recognize these so it attacks, which results in food sensitivities. You might not even be aware of these sensitivities, which can manifest as hives, allergies, chronic sinus inflammation, and migraines and become the triggers for irritable bowel syndrome and autoimmune disease.

HEALTHY GUT
versus LEAKY GUT

A healthy gut works like a cheesecloth, allowing only nutrients through, but keeping larger food particles and pathogenic bacteria, yeast, and parasites out. In a leaky gut, the tight junctions are loosened so undigested food particles and pathogens get through and activate the immune system, causing inflammation and food sensitivities.

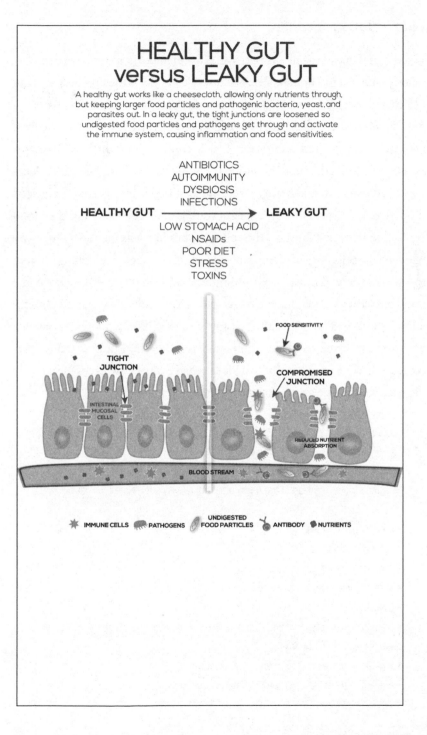

ANTIBIOTICS
AUTOIMMUNITY
DYSBIOSIS
INFECTIONS

HEALTHY GUT ———————→ **LEAKY GUT**

LOW STOMACH ACID
NSAIDs
POOR DIET
STRESS
TOXINS

TIGHT
JUNCTION

INTESTINAL
MUCOSAL
CELLS

FOOD SENSITIVITY

COMPROMISED
JUNCTION

REDUCED NUTRIENT
ABSORPTION

BLOOD STREAM

✳ IMMUNE CELLS 🦠 PATHOGENS ◯ UNDIGESTED FOOD PARTICLES Ⴤ ANTIBODY ◆ NUTRIENTS

Leaky Gut Syndrome

Leaky gut is one of the most controversial and important conditions to treat when looking at gut imbalances, because a leaky gut is the link between gut health and systemic illness. "Leaky gut" is not a diagnosis but a process, a description of the underlying pathology of numerous diseases that we treat yet have failed to find a cure for. It is a condition in which connections between the cells that line the inside of the intestines (known as *tight junctions*) become looser, allowing larger molecules (such as partially digested food particles) to pass through the gut wall. Usually, properly digested food is absorbed directly through the cell wall, but in a leaky gut, the pathway between the cells is opened up, exposing the gut-associated immune system to a wide variety of substances our immune cells would otherwise not come into contact with. Imagine a cheesecloth with a tight weave and one with a looser weave. The one with the tight weave will only allow the passage of liquids, minerals, and the components of digestion (amino acids, glucose, fats), whereas the one with a looser weave can allow pieces of partially digested food particles to escape through the gut lumen.

WHY DO PEOPLE DEVELOP A LEAKY GUT?

Many conditions may lead to the development of a leaky gut. This list includes:

- Poor dietary choices
- Stress/emotions
- Infections, including dysbiosis
- Systemic inflammatory diseases
- Low stomach acid
- Toxin exposure (preservatives and pesticides in foods may damage the lining, as well as environmental toxins)
- NSAIDs (like aspirin, ibuprofen, Advil, or Aleve)
- Antibiotics (with their disruption of normal gut flora)

Your immune system is constantly patrolling the gut border for anything it does not recognize in order to prevent an all-out invasion. As the immune system encounters these escaped particles, it attacks. And in individuals with a genetic predisposition to autoimmune diseases, this increased load on the immune system leads to the type of dysregulation that becomes an autoimmune disease. As you are exposed to large protein molecules in a leaky gut from the incompletely digested foods you eat on a daily basis, you develop immune reactions to those foods.

Common symptoms of this immune overactivation include:

- Bloating
- Indigestion
- Constipation/diarrhea
- Fatigue (through malnutrition)
- Weight gain (partly due to water retention)

Research has shown that IBS and migraines both can be triggered by the immune reactions to foods that a person may be consuming regularly. And if not treated, leaky gut can lead to many systemic inflammatory disorders and even malnutrition.

FOOD SENSITIVITIES EXPAND YOUR WAISTLINE

Often a diet rich in the foods that you are sensitive to, in combination with a leaky or *hyperpermeable* gut, leads to fluid retention and inflammation and, as a result, weight gain. People who are very food sensitive often lose five to six pounds in the first week after removing these foods from their diet.

You may be consuming foods that your body has developed an immune response or sensitivity to without your even knowing it. Even when you restrict yourself stringently by following one of the popular diets, including limiting calories or carbs, or monitoring carb-fat-protein ratios, your food sensitivities will make it very difficult to lose weight. When you remove the foods that are "toxic" to your body because they activate your immune response, weight loss happens naturally.

Gut Bacteria May Make You Fat

New evidence suggests that gut bacteria may alter the way fat is stored, the way hormones tell us we are full, and the way blood glucose levels are balanced. The wrong type of microbial diversity (or lack of diversity) can set the stage for obesity and its associated diseases, like diabetes and heart disease.

In one study, researchers took the gut microbes from four sets of human twins in which one twin was slim and the other obese and transferred them into two groups of mice. The mice had been raised in a germ-free environment (so their bodies would be free of any bacteria). The researchers found that the mice given microbes from an obese twin quickly gained weight, whereas the mice populated with microbes from the lean twin stayed thin. Both ate the same diet to factor out any differences in eating patterns as the reason for the weight gain.

When the researchers looked at the microbial populations from each of the human twins, they found the obese twins had a less diverse community of bacteria. Microbial diversity seems to be a key to health. Unfortunately, as the percentage of processed foods in our diets has increased over the last century, these foods have promoted in us less diverse gut microbial populations.

To see if obesity could be reversed simply by increasing the diversity of gut microbial population, thin mice were placed in the same cage with obese mice, and as a result of their comingling behavior the more diverse microbiota from the lean mice transferred to their obese cage mates, who had started with a less diverse population. This one-way transfer resulted in an improved metabolism and reversal of obesity in the obese mice. However, when fed a diet high in saturated fats, the obesity-prone mice gained weight and their bacterial flora remained less diverse.[3]

The ability to manipulate gut flora to affect weight in humans is still not as straightforward as it may seem in the mouse experiment above. Attempts to pinpoint which bacterial species are responsible for a normal body mass have yet to be successful. It is a very complex symbiotic system, but we do know it is affected by diet. A varied plant-based diet rich in whole foods stimulates the type of bacterial diversity that promotes weight loss, whereas a diet lacking this variety and full of processed foods will promote a less diverse population, which leads to weight gain.

FECAL TRANSPLANTATION FOR WEIGHT MANAGEMENT?

As research on the microbiome explodes, manipulation of the gut flora to effect changes in weight may be a possibility in the near future.

One pivotal study used fecal transplantation of intestinal microbiota from lean donors to overweight male recipients with metabolic syndrome—a condition characterized by weight gain and central obesity stemming from insulin resistance (more about this in Chapter 2). Six weeks after the fecal transplant, the insulin sensitivity of the male recipients improved (as measured through blood tests).[4] These studies are opening up the possibility of developing intestinal flora as therapeutic agents for metabolic syndrome and obesity.

Ultimately, understanding how the bacteria in our guts interact with one another will help us devise the types of therapies that create astonishing results by manipulating this previously underappreciated variable.

Gut-Associated Inflammation and Systemic Disease

As the gut-associated immune system becomes activated, it leads to a body-wide increased level of alertness, much like the U.S. terror alert. Messenger molecules secreted by our own immune cells result in inflammation, fat deposition in our bellies, weight gain, and systemic diseases. People who suffer from gut-associated inflammation will present with different symptoms. In one person, this inflammation can lead to migraines, asthma, or allergies; in another person, it can lead to an autoimmune disease. The individual expression is controlled by genes. However, underlying each of these potential outcomes is the same root cause: a gut system that was knocked out of balance and became inflamed. Anyone with an inflammatory chronic disease will benefit from an approach that takes into account the health of the gut.

Gut-Associated Inflammation and Cancer

Although cancer is a multifactorial disease, chronic inflammation and chronic activation of the immune system by certain infections are increasingly being recognized as important contributing factors.[5, 6] Here are some common associations:

- *H. pylori* infection and stomach MALT (mucosa-associated lymphoid tissue) lymphoma
- Schistosomiasis (a parasitic infection of the bladder) and bladder cancer
- Hepatitis B and C viruses and liver cancer

Among the top five most deadly cancers in the world, two are gastrointestinal. Stomach cancer is the third most common cause of cancer deaths worldwide, and the fourth most common is colon cancer.[7]

Cancer of the esophagus affects a minority of people in comparison but is also associated with chronic inflammation. Although smoking is a major risk factor, another important risk factor for esophageal cancer is acid reflux.[8] The reflux causes constant irritation and inflammation of the lower esophagus, leading to the changes in the cells that eventually become cancerous.

A major risk factor for colon cancer is inflammatory bowel disease, especially ulcerative colitis.[9] However, studies have also linked inflammation unrelated to IBD to colon cancer.[10]

GUT-ASSOCIATED INFLAMMATION AND BREAST CANCER

Some studies have suggested a possible association between gut inflammation and cancers outside of the gastrointestinal tract. One study looked at a possible link between prolonged gut inflammation and breast cancer.[11] The researchers discovered that mammary carcinoma developed within four to six weeks in mice that acquired an infection with *Helicobacter hepaticus,* a gut-associated pathogen. Perhaps gut bacteria should be on our radar when looking for the underlying causes of cancer.

Gut-Associated Inflammation and Pain

As we understand the association between gut inflammation and pain, more studies are supporting its role in arthritic conditions, such as spondyloarthropathies[12] (like ankylosing spondylitis) and rheumatoid arthritis. In addition, gut inflammation is associated with an even more common pain condition known as fibromyalgia, which affects up to 12 percent of the population.

In terms of pain disorders, fibromyalgia can be one of the most frustrating for both the patient and the health-care practitioner. It is a complex condition characterized by widespread musculoskeletal pain, fatigue, sleep disturbances, loss of memory, and depression. From my experience, I can tell you there is no one clear cause for fibromyalgia, and conventional treatments at best only manage symptoms but do not make the patient better. However, one piece of the puzzle that is often missed is a patient's gut health. Most have gut-associated inflammation. Working to address these gut issues—whether they are bacterial overgrowth, dysbiosis, or food sensitivities—often helps reduce overall body pain and improves these patients' general feelings of malaise.

Gabriella is an excellent example of this. When she came to see me for her unrelenting body pains, she already had a diagnosis of fibromyalgia from another doctor. As soon as I heard this, I dove into the details of her diet and lifestyle. Of note, she was eating a diet rich in sugar and processed carbohydrates and poor in inflammation-fighting omega-3s. I created an anti-inflammatory diet regimen for her that included avoiding sugar, wheat/gluten, corn, soy, and dairy and incorporated lots of vegetables and omega-3-rich foods. This was complemented by a supplement regimen designed to replenish healthy gut flora and reduce inflammation. After twenty-eight days on this program, Gabriella came back for a follow-up visit. She could not believe how much less swollen she felt with an amazing 50 percent reduction in her pain. After two years of suffering, Gabriella began to feel like her old self again. Her gut inflammation had been the fuel to the fire of her body pains. By beginning to put out the fire in her gut, we were able to reduce her total body pain.

In the case of my patient Julie, whom you met in the Introduction, with further questioning I noted that when she was in college, she often got strep throat, sinus infections, or urinary tract infections—between three and five times per year. She made multiple visits to the student health center and had been placed on multiple courses of antibiotics. Normally this would be a minor detail in a health history, except that when looking at the timeline of when her symptoms started and worsened, we see that the onset of her "irritable bowel" was during her last year in college.

We know that multiple courses of antibiotics destroy the intestinal flora—the "good" bacteria that live in our guts and help boost our immune system, produce vitamins for us (like vitamin K), and regulate critical elements of bowel function. Without the proper balance of good bacteria (known as probiotics, from the Latin *pro* and the Greek *biotic* meaning "for life"), the ecosystem is left wide open for predators to take over. Parasites, potentially pathogenic bacteria, and unfriendly yeast conquer the intestines. No wonder Julie was suffering from major gut *unhappiness*! She needed a gut reboot.

THE GUT C.A.R.E. PROGRAM

Behind my approach to all gut issues is what I call the Gut C.A.R.E. Program. C.A.R.E. stands for Cleanse, Activate, Restore, and Enhance. C.A.R.E. also stands for "caring" for your gut and yourself through a mind, body, and spirit approach. It is a gut "reboot" system designed to restore balance to the digestive tract and create total body wellness. No matter what the underlying imbalances are, the Gut C.A.R.E. Program gives you the template to follow to reestablish gut happiness. By following the Happy Gut Diet, balance is restored to the gut and inflammation is reversed. And, by fixing the gut, we accomplish much more than just a reduction in gut-associated inflammation; we fix inflammation everywhere in the body. By following the Gut C.A.R.E. Program, you can end systemic and abdominal pain, restore normal gut function, cleanse your body, lose weight, and regain energy. As a result, you will not only feel younger, but you will look younger, too.

C.A.R.E.

As an integrative physician, I believe in the innate ability of the body as a *whole* to heal itself when given the opportunity. Where balance has been lost, health can be restored by reestablishing equilibrium with an integrative, functional approach. I look at the body as a confluence of your mind, your physical self, and your spirit. To truly heal, you must address all three.

My passion for this approach inspired me to create my program for gut health known as the Gut C.A.R.E. Program.

CLEANSE	Remove gut irritants, infections, food sensitivities, and toxins in food
ACTIVATE	Reactivate healthy digestion by replacing essential nutrients and enzymes
RESTORE	Reintroduce beneficial bacteria for a healthy gut flora
ENHANCE	Repair, regenerate, and heal the intestinal lining

With the Gut C.A.R.E. Program you will heal your gut, get rid of bloating and gas, restore proper digestion, gain energy, and eliminate pain. Even better, improving your gut health will have beneficial repercussions for your entire body. Your skin will clear up, your mind will feel brighter and clearer, your allergies will disappear, and you will effortlessly lose weight.

This Functional Medicine approach to your health opens up a world of *answers* instead of a world of *classification*. With the proven Gut C.A.R.E. Program, you will not only become an expert on your gastrointestinal (GI) system, but you will be armed with the tools you need to end your gut-associated distress for good!

WHAT'S YOUR TIMELINE?

Of utmost importance behind every condition is the patient's story— your story. How did your symptoms come about? The timeline of how your symptoms started and progressed is *so* crucial to the Functional Medicine approach that I have included a downloadable timeline at www.happygutlife.com for you to fill out to help you clarify the time sequence of events that led to your symptoms. For example, did your symptoms start after a trip to a foreign country, where you may have picked up a parasite? Did your symptoms start or worsen after a round of antibiotics for recurrent sinus infections, or after several weeks of eating a diet high in simple carbohydrates? All of these details are clues as to where the problem may lie. When filling out your timeline, include as many health details as you can, even if they don't seem to be relevant. Include any medical intervention, including antibiotics taken for short or long durations. You can take your completed timeline to a Functional Medicine practitioner or naturopath and start working on the root causes of your condition(s). (Learn how to find a Functional Medicine practitioner in Appendix D: Resources.)

YOUR HEALTH EVENTS/SYMPTOM TIMELINE

The health events/symptom timeline is where you record key health events, like repeated courses of antibiotics for sinus or urinary tract infections, major infections, hospitalizations, and health events throughout your life and that immediately preceded the onset of your gut or gut-associated symptoms, even if they don't seem relevant to you. This is a great way to look for clues as to why your gut went out of balance and how you ended up with your current illness, whether it is fibromyalgia, lupus, migraines, chronic pain, or sudden weight gain. It's also a great tool to bring to your first visit with a Functional Medicine practitioner, because the story of how your symptoms evolved over time is very important in devising a treatment plan. See www.happygutlife.com for a downloadable version of the timeline.

BEFORE AND AFTER QUESTIONNAIRE

When my patients begin to feel better, they sometimes forget the details of how bad they felt in the beginning. Often, I have to remind them of the symptoms they reported at our first meeting. Recording your symptoms at this point will provide a reference and reminder of how your current way of living and eating is affecting your health. The Happy Gut Pre-Program Symptoms Questionnaire in the next pages will help you rate your symptom score now as a basis of comparison for after you complete the Gut C.A.R.E. Program. Base your answers on how you have generally felt over the thirty to ninety days prior to starting the program. This will be your pre-program symptom score. It is a great way to track your progress when you complete the Happy Gut Diet and Gut C.A.R.E. Program, and also a record of how you felt while it is fresh in your mind.

HAPPY GUT PRE-PROGRAM SYMPTOMS QUESTIONNAIRE

Rate each of the following symptoms based upon how you have felt over the past thirty to ninety days:

POINT SCALE

0   *Never* or *almost never* have the symptom

1   *Occasionally* have it, symptom is *not severe*

3   *Occasionally* have it, symptom is *severe*

5   *Frequently* have it, symptom is *not severe*

7   *Frequently* have it, symptom is *severe*

HEAD

___ Headaches/migraines

___ Light-headedness

___ Dizziness

___ Insomnia

Total _____

EYES

___ Watery, red, or itchy eyes

___ Swollen or sticky eyelids

___ Bags or dark circles under eyes

___ Blurred or tunnel vision (does not include near- or farsightedness)

Total _____

EARS

___ Itchy ears

___ Ear infections, earaches

___ Drainage from ear

___ Ringing in ears

Total _____

NOSE

___ Nasal congestion

___ Sinus problems

___ Runny nose

___ Sneezing attacks

___ Excessive mucus production

___ Frequent colds

Total _____

MOUTH/THROAT

___ Chronic cough

___ Frequently clearing throat of mucus

___ Sore throat, hoarseness, loss of voice

___ Swollen, pale, and/or red tongue or gums

___ White, frothy coating on tongue

___ Canker sores or mouth ulcers

Total _____

GUT

___ Nausea, vomiting

___ Diarrhea

___ Constipation

___ Bloated feeling

___ Excessive belching, passing gas

___ Heartburn

___ Abdominal pain

Total _____

SKIN

___ Acne

___ Hives, rashes, eczema

___ Hair loss or thinning hair

___ Flushing, hot flashes

___ Excessive sweating

Total _____

CHEST/HEART

___ Irregular or skipped heartbeat

___ Rapid or pounding heartbeat after eating

___ Chest pain after or between meals

Total _____

LUNGS

___ Chest tightness or congestion

___ Asthma, wheezing, or bronchitis

___ Shortness of breath

___ Difficulty breathing with exertion

Total _____

GENITAL/URINARY

___ Frequent or urgent urination

___ Difficulty urinating

___ Penile itching or discharge

___ Vaginal itching or discharge

Total _____

JOINTS/MUSCLE

___ Painful, swollen, or achy joints

___ Arthritis

___ Stiffness or limitation of movement

___ Painful or achy muscles

___ Feeling of weakness or fatigue

Total _____

WEIGHT

___ Excessive eating/drinking

___ Craving certain foods (like bread or desserts)

___ Excessive weight gain

___ Compulsive eating

___ Water retention

___ Unexpected weight loss

Total _____

ENERGY/ACTIVITY

___ Fatigue, sluggishness

___ Lethargy, lack of motivation to move

___ Excessive energy

___ Agitation

Total _____

MIND

___ Memory loss

___ Confusion, poor comprehension

___ Mental fog

___ Poor concentration

___ Poor balance

___ Indecisiveness

___ Word-finding difficulties

___ Difficulty learning

Total _____

EMOTIONS

___ Mood swings

___ Anxiety, fear, nervousness

___ Anger, irritability, aggressiveness

___ Depression

Total _____

GRAND TOTAL ____

Each individual score can help you determine your trouble spots. The total score is a baseline for comparison with your score at the end of the program.

At the end of the program you will fill out the same questionnaire, the Post-Program Symptoms Questionnaire, in Appendix B. I want you to fill it out based on how you feel at the end of the twenty-eight-day Gut C.A.R.E. Program and Happy Gut Diet. Compare your individual and total scores. What improved? What still needs improvement?

2

THE HAPPY GUT DIET:
PHASE I EXPLAINED

NOW THAT YOU HAVE an overview of the Gut C.A.R.E. Program and how gut-related issues can affect your entire body, let's look in detail at each of the foods or food additives you will avoid for the next twenty-eight days as part of Phase I of the Happy Gut Diet. I want you to better understand why these foods are making you sick and leaving you toxic and overweight and feeling zapped of energy.

SUGAR IS YOUR TRIGGER

When Leslie came to see me, she was suffering from sporadic joint inflammation and random low-grade fevers, and her hands and feet were puffy and swollen. She ached all over and had seen multiple doctors, and no one could figure out what was going on with her. She had been tested for all sorts of infectious diseases, including Lyme disease and rheumatoid arthritis, but all the markers were negative. So she'd been given the default diagnosis of "fibromyalgia"—an umbrella term used to describe her array of symptoms without explaining the cause, as Western medicine often does. None of the classic medications—like Cymbalta, an antidepressant, or Lyrica, a nerve pain modifier with horrible side effects—reduced her pain, discomfort, and general malaise. When going over her history, I noted that her diet was rich in sugar. She could not resist the temptation to eat candies commonly kept around her office; while at home, ice cream, cakes, and other desserts were the norm rather than the exception. Delving deeper into her sugar addiction, I noted how her high-stress job triggered her cravings. She was seeing me for acupuncture to manage the stress; however, we started talking about all of her health issues, and it was immediately obviously that sugar was causing her major problems.

Sugar may be a culprit in:

- Depression
- Mood swings
- Irritability
- Symptoms of premenstrual syndrome
- Menopausal hot flashes
- Migraines
- "Fibromyalgia"
- Body aches and pains
- Heart disease
- Diabetes
- Vascular disease

By sugar, I mean refined cane sugar, but it can also mean high-fructose corn syrup (HFCS—more about this later) or any other sweetening derivatives. When you ingest too much sugar, it's like you just boarded a roller coaster—you better buckle up, because you're about to go for a ride. Initially, sugar satisfies the craving centers in the brain, increases your blood pressure and heart rate, and can give you the feeling of an energy surge. Soon your insulin levels start to rise to stabilize and control the blood sugar level, and as a result your blood sugar begins to drop, and you start to feel irritable, angry, and easily provoked. Your patience wears thin. You then start to feel drowsy, tired, perhaps slightly headachy or with pressure in your sinuses. If you're particularly toxic, you can feel the effects in your muscles and joints. Then, about one to two hours after you had the sugar-rich snack, your sugar drops low enough that your body has to kick into high gear. Cortisol is secreted to now stabilize your blood sugar and maintain homeostasis (a balanced environment). The high cortisol is a stress to your adrenals, and it winds you up. You may feel panicky, anxious, and unsettled. Soon your brain is telling you it wants another hit. Yes, that's right—sugar is like a drug to your brain. As your blood sugar drops, you will crave more of it to keep you near the high.

The problem is that the "sugar-coaster" keeps going up and then crashing down. The more you do, the harder you fall.

My sugar-addicted patients can live their entire day on the sugar-coaster. Another patient, Angelique, had a psychological and behavioral addiction to sugar—exacerbated by stress!

Angelique had a high-level position, answering directly to the CEO. Her profession was marked by deadlines that consumed all of her time, leaving no opportunities for self-care. She added to that by holding herself up to a very high standard while also being the person whom everyone went to with their problems. She had a tough time creating healthy boundaries—she couldn't say no to others. She couldn't say no to sugar, either. It was this level of perfection with no escape—except for the doughnut, cookie, or pastry whenever she found herself in a stressful event—that led her to put on more than fifty pounds of excess weight. This behavior had become so automatic that she didn't even realize (until we started talking about it) that she was instantly reaching for a candy bar or cookie the minute her stress levels shot through the roof. The trigger was always a stressful event. Her coping mechanism was to reach for sweets.

Even though a habitual behavior like this is difficult to break, once she recognized this unconscious behavior, she was able to take a step back and realize how damaging it was. As with Leslie, the sugar caused Angelique's body to swell up, and although no one had diagnosed her with "fibromyalgia," she lived with fatigue, body aches, and general malaise.

When it comes to sugar, the hardest thing to overcome is the individual reason why it has become compulsive for you. What are you self-treating through your sugar addiction? Look at your reasons for eating and craving sugar. Do you find yourself reaching for a sweet when you're under duress? Do you crave sugar when you feel your life is not going the way you want it to go? Do you associate a bar of milk chocolate or a box of cookies with a reward for yourself after a hard day at the office? As a child, did your parents use sugar as a reward for good behavior? These are all reasons someone might reach for a sugar-laden snack, like eating ice cream in front of the TV at night or late-night snacking in the kitchen.

And it's not all your fault! Sugar is highly addictive. A study using rats showed that sugar is more addictive than cocaine—one of the most addictive substances known. When given a choice between the two, the cocaine-addicted rats switched to sugar water.[1] But don't give up hope, because you can easily detox from added sugar in your diet, and the Gut C.A.R.E. Program is designed to help you do just that.

TEN REASONS SUGAR IS BAD FOR YOU

1. **Sugar is unsustainable energy** and devoid of essential minerals, vitamins, essential fatty acids, or protein.
2. **Sugar is linked to a decrease in the intake of essential micronutrients.** When you eat sugar, you're less likely to enjoy nutrient-packed foods because they will taste bland. You'll feel so full from sugar-dense foods that you won't want to eat foods in the phytonutrient spectrum.
3. **Cane sugar is high in fructose,** and it's a fifty-fifty mixture of glucose and fructose. Fructose can overload the liver, which is the only place in the body that can metabolize it. Fructose also does not turn off the hunger hormone, ghrelin, making you eat more.
4. **Too much sugar (including HFCS) can lead to a fatty liver.** Along with worldwide obesity, fatty liver is a growing problem and can lead to metabolic disease and fibrosis of the liver.

5. **Sugar can cause insulin resistance,** which can lead to metabolic syndrome, a major cause of heart and vascular disease, and diabetes, a major cause of health problems that destroy quality of life.

6. **Sugar causes inflammation,** and inflammation leads to pain.

7. **Sugar is linked to an increase in body weight in both children and adults.** Sugar is a major contributor to the rising rates of obesity across all age groups.

8. **Sugar is highly addictive.** Sugar leads to dopamine release in the brain, which makes eating it feel rewarding.

9. **Sugar feeds cancer.** People who eat excessive sugar are at a higher risk of getting cancer.

10. **Sugar raises your cholesterol.** It's not the fat in your diet that's raising your cholesterol; it's the sugar.

What About Sugar Substitutes?

Sugar substitutes, the so-called artificial sugars, are no better. They are found in products like Crystal Light and diet sodas. How many sugar-free drinks or diet sodas have you drunk because you believed: 1) they would help you lose weight, 2) they tasted better than water, and 3) they were better for you than sugar-laden sodas or alternative drinks? These sugar substitutes are just as bad for your waistline and may even be worse. According to research, drinkers of diet sodas experience a 70 percent greater increase in waist circumference than nonusers. And shockingly, those who drank two or more diet sodas a day saw their waists increase by 500 percent more than nonusers![2]

But wait—if that's not enough, the artificial sweeteners in diet sodas increase your risk of stroke, heart attack, metabolic syndrome, and cardiovascular disease.[3] Is that enough information to get you to stop drinking these artificially sweetened drinks today?

SIX REASONS TO NEVER DRINK A DIET BEVERAGE AGAIN

1. They actually make you gain weight.
2. They increase your risk of stroke, heart attack, metabolic syndrome, and cardiovascular disease.
3. They overstimulate your sweet receptors so you cannot appreciate the natural sweetness in foods (like berries).
4. Phosphoric acid in diet sodas leaches calcium from your bones, which can lead to weak bones and fractures.
5. Aspartame, an artificial sweetener, is a neurotoxin.
6. The caramel color in sodas, created by 4-methylimidazole (4-MEI), is a known carcinogen.

SAY GOOD-BYE TO GLUTEN

Often when I tell my patients that they will have to avoid gluten (wheat), they look at me like a deer caught in the headlights. They all seem to respond the same way, asking, "What do I eat now?" For anyone who is used to having an abundance of wheat (like bread, pasta, and other flour-containing products) in his or her diet, it can be like taking away a child's favorite toy. That's because wheat is addictive. A protein from gluten, *gliadorphin*, interacts with opiate receptors in the brain, mimicking the effects of opiate drugs like heroin and morphine.[4] These compounds affect the temporal lobe—an area in the brain that is associated with speech and hearing comprehension. This is why you can feel cloudy-headed after a hefty dose of bread.

When John came to see me, he was struggling with a twenty-pound weight gain, recurrent sinus infections, nasal polyps, and constant nasal congestion. He had been working with an ear, nose, and throat specialist and had been placed on multiple courses of antibiotics. When I first examined him, his nasal passages were inflamed and full of tiny bumps known as polyps. Polyps are believed to be caused by an allergic response, most likely to airborne allergens.

Even the changes that I identified in his nasal mucosa are traditionally associated with a condition termed "allergic rhinitis," which describes the inflammatory response inside the nose to environmental allergens. What is often missed is that the allergy may not be coming from the outside world. In John's case, it had to do with an internal reaction to a food he was ingesting on a regular basis. I had a strong suspicion that his issue was food. As part of his evaluation, I tested him for gluten sensitivity, along with sensitivities to other foods. It was no surprise to me that he came back strongly positive for a wheat/gluten sensitivity. I prescribed a gluten-free diet.

John writes, "The idea of eliminating gluten from my diet was very intimidating to me. I was something of a bread junkie—I loved it in all its forms. So even as Dr. Pedre was outlining the ways the diet could help me, in my mind I was searching for ways not to lose my morning bagel. 'I think what I'll do is cut out pasta first,' I told him. 'Then work on sandwiches, then move on to . . .' Dr. Pedre quickly responded that I would make it harder on myself by doing it that way. He suggested I go cold turkey instead. To really see the results I'd get from avoiding gluten, I'd have to go 100 percent."

One month later, I saw John for a follow-up. He came in reporting a weight loss of ten pounds with less nasal congestion and sinus pressure. He told me he realized that once he had changed his mental programming about what he ate and how to replace gluten in his meals with whole foods, including vegetables and protein, the new diet was actually not that difficult to follow. The immediate improvements motivated him to continue the program. Three months later, he returned with the amazing report that his nasal polyps, which the ENT had wanted to remove surgically, were receding with the dietary changes. He had lost the twenty pounds he had been struggling with and had been able to start exercising again.

Gluten is a sticky protein that gives bread products their fluffiness and chewiness. These are such desirable traits that the food industry has hybridized the wheat plant to have 30 to 50 percent more gluten than it did half a century ago. Not only does it save in raw material for food production, but it gives these foods the characteristics that we find pleasing, like the lightness and porousness of a "risen" bread. Unfortunately, for many people it poses a real problem.

Gluten is actually made up of two proteins: *glutenins* and *gliadins*. When people are sensitive to gluten, they may be having a reaction to one of these proteins or to one of their breakdown subunits, which leads to inflammation. Because of this, it is often difficult to diagnose gluten sensitivity. Most routine laboratory tests do not test for all of these proteins. (See Appendix D: Resources for laboratories that can test for all of these proteins.)

How Big Is This Problem?

It is estimated that between 10 and 30 percent of the U.S. population has a sensitivity to gluten, and 2 percent of the population has celiac disease. Most have no idea they are sensitive. This is caused by immune reactions that occur in response to any of a number of gluten metabolites and gluten-related proteins. In the case of full-blown celiac disease, an autoimmune reaction resulting from the gliadin component of gluten leads to body-wide inflammation. This inflammation may be expressed in a variety of ways in different people:

- Obesity
- Weight gain
- Difficulty losing weight
- Lack of mental clarity
- Inability to focus
- Extreme fatigue
- Inability to put on weight
- Diarrhea or constipation
- Skin rashes (like dermatitis herpetiformis)

- Muscle pain
- Headaches (like migraines)

Many doctors don't believe that gluten sensitivity exists outside of the diagnosis of full-blown celiac disease. However, new research is showing that people can become sensitive to gluten without developing autoimmune celiac disease.

Although there are tests available to determine gluten sensitivity (see Chapter 6), the best test is removing gluten from the diet and monitoring for the changes that occur. The minimum time to note changes is at least two weeks, but the changes in your health will be more apparent to you after four weeks. When changes happen slowly over days, sometimes it's hard to notice until the difference in your symptoms is large enough to catch your attention. My patients are often amazed, however, by how quickly they feel less swollen and less bloated as their bodies detox from gluten—and within just two weeks! The good news is that even those with severe gluten sensitivity will experience benefits in the long run. Patience, determination, and consistency are the keys to success.

Hidden Gluten

Gluten is not only found in wheat. There are a variety of gluten-containing grains and foods, namely barley, bulgur, couscous, farro, graham, kamut, oats,[5] orzo, rye, semolina, spelt, and triticale. As you can see, gluten may actually be hidden in a number of foods you eat regularly without your even knowing it's there. It is often used to help thicken sauces and gravies or in the preparation of meatballs and burgers (like turkey), which is something to be aware of when eating out. A friend of mine with a severe gluten intolerance was told her meal was gluten-free, when in fact she ended up having a gluten reaction thirty-six hours later. When she called to speak to the restaurant's chef, she found out that the turkey burger she had eaten was prepared with bread crumbs in order to give it more volume and keep it from crumbling apart. A food preparation trick left her sick for a couple of days. Thankfully, more and more restaurants and food establishments are becoming sensitive to the reactions people may have to gluten and are helping people know which foods contain gluten with simple labeling. But not all products that contain gluten are labeled as such. Not only is gluten found in processed foods, but it also is added to personal care products, such as makeup, shampoos, and conditioners. You can thank gluten for that "volumizing" hair conditioner! While it's sitting on your scalp softening your hair, your body absorbs some of that gluten through your scalp. And if you are particularly sensitive, even this small amount of exposure can lead to inflammation in distant areas inside your body.

GLUTEN-FREE GRAINS, FLOURS, AND STARCHES	GLUTEN-CONTAINING GRAINS, FLOURS, AND STARCHES
Amaranth	Barley
Arrowroot	Bulgur
Bean flours (garbanzo, fava, Romano)	Cakes
Buckwheat	Cereals
Corn	Chapati flour (atta)
Fava beans	Dinkel
Flaxseed	Durum
Garbanzo beans (chickpeas)	Einkorn
Garfava flour (garbanzo and fava bean)	Emmer
Hominy	Farina
Mesquite flour	Farro, fu
Millet	Graham flour
Montina flour	Kamut
Nut flour and nut meals	Malt (extract, flavoring, syrup, vinegar)
Oats (uncontaminated with gluten)	Oats (commercial brands, oat bran, or syrup)
Pea flour	Orzo
Potato flour or potato starch	Rye
Quinoa	

GLUTEN-FREE GRAINS, FLOURS, AND STARCHES	GLUTEN-CONTAINING GRAINS, FLOURS, AND STARCHES
Rice, all forms	Semolina
Rice bran	Spelt
Sago	Textured vegetable protein
Sorghum flour	Triticale
Soy flour	Wheat bran, germ, or starch
Tapioca (manioc, cassava, yucca)	
Teff flour	

Many people who lack gastrointestinal symptoms when they eat wheat or gluten are actually suffering from an assault on their bodies without realizing it, often involving their joints, muscles, and nervous system. When the immune system becomes activated by gluten or one of its metabolites, it sends out messages that tell your body to create inflammation in distant regions as a response to an onslaught of food proteins that have been classified as enemies of the body. When you continuously eat these foods, you may register only a general feeling of malaise and not be able to pinpoint any specific body symptom. However, once you completely eliminate the food from your diet and become symptom-free, then reintroduce the food a couple of weeks or months later, suddenly very specific symptoms, like a sinus headache or joint swelling, come back. Eureka! You can then make the association between eating that food and the random set of symptoms you used to have all the time.

Gluten also hides in the following:

Baked beans

Blue cheese

Bran flakes

Brown rice syrup

Chocolate

Couscous

Fake crabmeat

Gravies and sauces

Hydrolyzed veggie protein

Pâtés

Pumpernickel

Salad dressings

Sausages	Soy sauce
Seitan (pure gluten!)	Spice blends
Soups	

It is no surprise that even the most reluctant to give up bread and pasta become the strongest advocates for a gluten-free diet when they experience the remarkable benefits themselves.

More Reasons to Not Eat Gluten

Even though gluten gets all the bad press these days, these two accomplices can be just as damaging. *Lectins* and *phytates* are antinutrients found in all gluten-containing grains. Lectins are also found in beans (they are particularly high in red kidney beans), dairy, and the nightshade vegetables (tomatoes, eggplant, peppers, and potatoes).

Lectins are sugar-binding proteins and, like gluten, are very sticky molecules. Their complexity makes them resistant to digestion, even to stomach acid, which allows them to enter our bloodstream unchanged. That's where they cause some real damage. Once absorbed, lectins can bind to many tissues, including in the thyroid and pancreas, and to the collagen in our joints. They then attract white blood cells to these tissues, potentially leading to an autoimmune response.[6] Lectins may be involved in the pathogenesis of diabetes, autoimmune thyroiditis, and rheumatoid arthritis. And lectin-containing foods may actually be at the root of chronic pain syndromes that many people suffer from.

Remember insulin, the very important blood sugar–regulating hormone? Lectins block insulin receptors so that they cannot receive the signal from your very own insulin. This leads to the much-dreaded insulin resistance, which causes your body to require more insulin to balance the same amount of sugar in the blood and leads to fat accumulation around the middle, weight gain, obesity, and eventually diabetes. Instead, we want less insulin circulating, lower blood sugar fluctuations, and to know when to stop eating.

And speaking of weight loss . . .

The other problem with lectins is that they lead to *leptin resistance*. *Leptin* is a very important hormone that regulates feelings of fullness. The more leptin in circulation, the less hungry you should be. However, the brains of people who are obese do not respond to the leptin signal. Their levels are high, but these levels are not sensed by their brain to signal that they are full and they should stop eating. Thus lectins lead to leptin resistance, leaving you hungry when you've already had all the food you need.

Because they are so sticky, lectins can also bind to our gut lining. This interferes with our normal gut flora and also contributes to gut hyperpermeability—or a leaky gut—by poking holes in our intestines that allow large undigested food proteins to enter our bloodstream. This sets off an inflammatory response that leads to a host of problems discussed previously. Basically, when we are internally inflamed, more of the calories that we eat are stored as fat and weight gain occurs.

As if that isn't enough, lectins stimulate the release of histamine in our stomachs, leading to acid hypersecretion. I have found that patients who suffer from acid reflux benefit from a gluten-free, grain-reduced diet. I have seen patients suffering from unrelenting reflux symptoms improve completely with these dietary changes and no medications.

Because lectins are so resistant to stomach acid and our own digestive enzymes, the best protection against them is to not eat them.

Phytates, another antinutrient, are just as bad as lectins. They interfere with the absorption of important minerals like calcium, iron, magnesium, copper, and zinc. All along we have been told to consume whole grains to get a healthy dose of vitamins and minerals. But consuming wheat, for example, can actually block calcium absorption in the long term, leading to osteoporosis.

PHYTATES: THE ANTINUTRIENT

Otherwise known as phytic acid, phytates are found in all gluten-containing grains as well as the outer coating of seeds and nuts. One way to counter their antinutrient effects is to consume sprouted grains. Nuts and seeds can be soaked overnight, then rinsed before using them in recipes or for eating. You can find delicious sprouted or presoaked nuts and seeds in specialty health-food stores. In Phase I of the Happy Gut Diet, a small amount of gluten-free grains, such as rice, millet, buckwheat, oats, and amaranth, is allowed.

Gluten and Thyroid Disease

Not enough reasons to make the jump to a gluten-free diet? Then consider that gluten may be slowing down your metabolism. It can actually interfere with your thyroid function, leading to autoimmune thyroid disease, weight gain, and difficulty losing weight.

Gluten in the body can also pose a case of mistaken identity. You see, the 3-D structure of gliadin, the main protein in gluten, looks a lot like thyroid proteins. When a person has a leaky gut and eats gluten, and gliadin makes it through the holes in the intestinal cell tight junctions, the immune system identifies this protein as a foreign substance and tags it for attack. But once the body has mounted an attack against gliadin, it can get confused through this molecular mimicry and start attacking the thyroid gland. This means that if you have autoimmune thyroid disease, like

Hashimoto's or Grave's disease, when you eat gluten your body will also attack your thyroid. Having Hashimoto's is like having a slow-burning fire in your thyroid. How do you put out this fire? Stop eating gluten (along with soy—more about that later).

Even more bad news: each time you eat gluten, the immune response it triggers can last up to six months. So there is no cheating when it comes to autoimmune thyroid disease and gluten. You've got to cut it out 100 percent if you're serious about helping your thyroid recover. I see patients every week who have normal thyroid function tests but test positive for thyroid antibodies. This means that even if they are not showing symptoms yet, they will eventually if they don't make the dietary changes today that will improve the health of their thyroid glands tomorrow.

Don't Fall into the Gluten-Free Trap

I've been talking about how gluten is bad for you and how great it is to go on a gluten-free diet. But there is one pitfall: the gluten-free aisle at your local supermarket. Just because something is labeled as gluten-free doesn't mean it is automatically healthier for you. Although it's great to have all this variety, you must be wary of substituting everything you used to eat that was wheat based with its gluten-free cousin.

The problem comes back to sugar. Often, gluten-free products are overly processed, and they usually are full of refined carbs. For example, a gluten-free slice of bread made from rice, tapioca, and almond flours can be just as bad as a slice of white bread because of its strong glycemic[7] effects (raising your blood sugar). To make matters even more complicated, the commonly found gluten substitute—corn—has proteins with amino acid sequences that look like gluten proteins. New science is even revealing that these gluten-like proteins in corn have led to an immune reaction in patients with celiac disease.[8]

While I'm steering you away from gluten, I am also directing you to eat whole foods, including lean or healthy fat proteins, slow carbs, non-starchy vegetables, nuts, and seeds. If you fill up with gluten-free substitutes, you are eating what I call "sugar equivalents" (SE) because the starches in these products break down to glucose (a component of sugar) through digestion. In effect, you are continuing to feed your sugar addiction. While believing that you have made healthy changes in your diet, you will not see the changes in your waistline. In fact, gluten-free substitutes can have the same effect on insulin as all other glucose-containing carbs, and you could end up putting on even more weight.

Don't forget the best gluten-free alternatives come from the earth. Included in my list of favorites are avocados, arugula, artichokes, all varieties of berries, baby romaine, and sweet potatoes. I do also enjoy a gluten-free pasta on occasion, but this is the exception rather than the rule. For now, while you're losing the gut, make it a point to not overindulge in gluten-free substitutes. Make them a small side, if that, but not the main focus of your meals.

DROP THE DAIRY

When Sonia came in to see me, she was in continuous intestinal distress. Her symptoms alternated between constipation and diarrhea. Her digestive system seemed to have a mind of its own. She also suffered from fatigue that worsened as the day went on. By the time she was done with work as a schoolteacher in the early afternoon, she could barely keep her eyes open. When I asked her about her diet, she said she tried to eat as healthy as possible. Every morning she had a Greek yogurt with a banana or berries and a coffee with a small amount of half-and-half. She ate salads for lunch, snacked on cheese and vegetables, and tried to make homemade meals with a protein, a starch, and a veggie side dish for dinner most nights of the week. What she thought was healthy (that is, yogurt, cheese, and dairy) for her was actually causing damage.

Milk contains two main proteins: *casein* and *whey*. Homogenized, pasteurized milk is devoid of the enzymes that help baby cows digest and utilize these proteins. For many people these proteins are hard to digest and can lead to food sensitivities. In addition, milk contains a sugar known as *lactose,* which is actually composed of two sugars—a glucose plus a *galactose.* Many people lack sufficient quantity of the enzyme *lactase* to break down lactose into its component parts, which are easier to absorb. This type of deficiency leads to an intolerance to milk that causes symptoms of gas, bloating, and diarrhea as the bacteria in the human gut ferment the lactose sugar instead.

Lactose intolerance is different from a food sensitivity, as its effects can be felt from almost immediately to within thirty to sixty minutes following a meal, and it is not immune mediated. Anyone who suffers from lactose intolerance will tell you how painful and uncomfortable it can be.

Sonia's primary problem was lactose intolerance. When I explained to her how dairy may actually be damaging to her intestinal lining and causing the wrong types of bacteria to overgrow, she understood and followed my prescription for a dairy-free diet; we also removed gluten. By the time we met for a follow-up four weeks later, she was eating a better balance of protein and vegetables with no dairy. Her bloating, diarrhea, and constipation had mostly resolved, and she was starting to feel a renewed level of energy, even in the afternoon when she used to experience a slump. She was so encouraged that she chose to continue on a dairy-free diet for a couple of months to solidify the positive changes.

WHAT ARE THE BEST MILK ALTERNATIVES?

- **Soy milk?** No way, Jose!!! (See more on page 62.)
- **Rice milk.** Beware—some brands may have gluten. Also, it's another grain, and we want to limit these, even rice.

- **Nut milks,** such as almond and cashew. The best ones are homemade. In store-bought brands look for the unsweetened variety and avoid those containing carrageenan.*
- **Coconut milk.** Nutrient packed, but avoid any in-store brands with carrageenan.*
- **Hemp milk.** Derived from hemp seeds, a great source of omega-3 fats. But watch out for added sugar.

*Carrageenan, a red-seaweed derivative, is a common ingredient added to commercially produced almond and coconut milks (among other products) as a thickener to improve texture. It is under debate as to whether it is safe for consumption if you have bowel issues like IBS or inflammatory bowel disease. Research shows that it is not safe. In fact, it can lead to gut inflammation. It is best to avoid it when you can. It may even be found in products labeled "organic."

Why Is Bovine Growth Hormone Bad?

If you think the benefits of a dairy-free diet apply only to the gut, think again. A dairy-free diet can give you healthy, vibrant, glowing skin. In another patient, we uncovered that a major culprit underlying her adult acne was dairy. Mass-produced dairy has higher levels of hormones like recombinant bovine growth hormone (rBGH or also rBST), which is a hormone injected into lactating cows to keep them producing milk by promoting growth of the mammary glands.

When pharmaceutical giant Genentech discovered and patented the gene for bovine growth hormone in the 1970s, it began looking for ways it could reproduce the gene using recombinant DNA technology. Genentech devised a way to hijack the DNA machinery of a bacterium like *E. coli* and make it produce this hormone. By 1981, the first trials of rBGH on cattle were complete, and by 1986, the U.S. Food and Drug Administration (FDA) had approved its use, deeming the consumption of food from rBGH-treated cows to be "safe." However, other countries have disagreed on its safety. rBGH has been banned in Canada, Japan, Australia, and all twenty-eight countries of the European Union.

Milk from cows treated with rBGH contains higher levels of BGH and insulin-like growth factor 1 (IGF-1), a hormone that can lead to low blood sugar. Even more concerning is IGF-1's possible role in increasing the risk of colon, breast, and prostate cancer. Research has found that in genetically susceptible men and women over the age of forty, IGF-1 can promote tumor growth. Do you really need more of this hormone circulating in your body from drinking milk?

DOES MILK REALLY DO A BODY GOOD?

Do you also believe that dairy is keeping your bones strong? If this were the case, why is dairy consumption the highest in the Western world, where the rates of osteoporosis also happen to be the highest? In his book *The China Study,* Dr. T. Colin Campbell writes:

> *Protein and even calcium—when consumed at excessive levels—are capable of increasing the risk of osteoporosis. Dairy, unfortunately, is the only food that is rich in both of these nutrients. Hegsted, backed by his . . . calcium research, said in his 1986 paper, " . . . hip fractures are more frequent in populations where dairy products are commonly consumed and calcium intakes are relatively high." Years later, the dairy industry still suggests . . . its products to build strong bones and teeth. The confusion, conflict and controversy [are] rampant . . .[9]*

Dairy Products Are Addictive

To my shock and dismay, the dairy industry has even petitioned the FDA to allow it to change the definition of dairy to include dairy products that are artificially sweetened—without having to mention the added sweetener on the label. The dairy industry wanted to make its products (like chocolate milk in school cafeterias) taste sweeter so kids would want to consume more of them. Not only is this appalling because of the information we have about artificial sweeteners, but it is also deceptive, misleading, and downright wrong! Artificial sweeteners have no place in foods consumed by children and teenagers, especially with our knowledge of their role in expanding waistlines and the already rising rates of obesity in this group. The way dairy is going, it will make you even fatter. And there is another problem with dairy.

The same way that gluten metabolizes into an opiate-like substance, so does the protein casein found in milk and other dairy products. Casein also has an opiate-like metabolite that can have the same effect as opium or morphine on the brain. This metabolite is known as *casomorphin*. Just like morphine, it makes you feel calmer, sleepier, and slightly elated. Your brain loves it, and so do you. Casein is not only found in dairy products but is often added to protein bars and protein shakes. It may even be found in whey protein (another milk protein) products, even if it is unlisted.

COMMON FOODS WHERE DAIRY MAY BE HIDING

Baked goods (cakes, cookies, scones, muffins)
Canned foods
Chocolate (except pure cocoa chocolates)
Eggs Benedict
Margarine
Mashed potatoes
Pancakes
Salad dressings (again, read labels! Or better yet, make your own)
Sauces (in restaurants)
Soups and chowders (with cream)
Waffles
Whey protein supplements

The whole foods in the Happy Gut Diet will give your body the calcium it needs. By avoiding grains containing gluten, you will not be consuming phytates that interfere with the absorption of calcium. You will get more nutrients from eating less food. In other words, without counting calories, you will naturally consume more nutrient-dense foods and fewer calorie-dense foods. Your body will respond positively by restoring itself to balance through the reduction in inflammation created by removing dairy and the other high-sensitivity foods from your diet.

WHEY: A HEALTHY NUTRITIONAL SUPPLEMENT?

Whey is a by-product of the manufacturing of cultured dairy products like cheese and yogurt. Whey has become a predominant nutritional supplement in protein drinks used by bodybuilders and athletes. Not all whey extraction processes create a pure product. If you are drinking whey for its health benefits, make sure that it is a *whey isolate,* or even better yet a *whey protein hydrolysate.* The whey protein hydrolysate, which involves another manufacturing step that makes it more expensive, delivers predigested whey protein that is easier for your digestive tract to break down and absorb. *Whey protein concentrates* will still be contaminated with casein, and for this reason people sensitive to dairy will experience a lot of the same symptoms of bloating, gas, and diarrhea. Therefore, read your labels, and know what you are consuming.

THE GOOD AND BAD ABOUT EGGS

Eggs are among the top ten food allergens. Many people develop a sensitivity to eggs over their lives. They may react to the egg yolk, the egg white, or both. Eggs also happen to be a pro-inflammatory food. Now, not all inflammation is bad, as we need inflammation to fight off infections and protect injured areas in the body, but too much inflammation, especially internal inflammation created by our diets, is bad for us. The key is having the right balance of anti-inflammatory omega-3s and pro-inflammatory omega-6s. Ideally, you want your body to be able to turn inflammation on and off as needed. You don't want inflammation to go on and on unchecked as it often does with the pro-inflammatory Standard American Diet.

Egg yolk is high in *arachidonic acid* (AA), a compound that is used in metabolic pathways that promote inflammation. AA is a source of omega-6 fatty acids that provide the body with messenger molecules (for example, leukotrienes, prostaglandins, prostacyclins, and thromboxanes) involved in the inflammatory response. For this reason, egg yolks are not part of an anti-inflammatory diet.

Egg yolks are not the only food high in AA; so are corn and corn-fed beef. Mass-produced corn-fed beef is full of pro-inflammatory omega-6s, whereas grass-fed beef is instead full of *inflammation-reducing* omega-3s. (For an in-depth look at the beef industry, read Michael Pollan's book *The Omnivore's Dilemma*.) Just like with meat, when we eat eggs from hens fed an unnatural diet based on soy and corn, we are basically consuming these food allergens indirectly. Mass-produced eggs come from hens raised on foods that were not natural or typical parts of their evolutionary diets. That's not good for the hens, and it's not good for us!

Organic eggs from cage-free hens fed a natural, free-range diet rich in omega-3s are much better for us, and they are allowed after the twenty-eight-day Elimination Phase of the Happy Gut Diet. The best eggs are locally sourced at a farmers' market, where you can speak to the farmer and find out how the hens are raised. Again, do your research. Don't just know *what* you are eating, know *where* what you are eating came from and, whenever possible, what *it* ate.

SO LONG, SOY

Soy and soy derivatives have infiltrated all corners of our food supply. From tofu to edamame to less obvious places like protein bars and powders, nutritional supplements, ice cream, cheeses, and chocolate (added as soy lecithin or simply lecithin), soy is everywhere. The American Heart Association has even adopted soy as the new heart-healthy alternative, based on some evidence that it helps lower cholesterol. But the products that tout the American Heart Association "healthy heart" symbol are often processed cereals and soy milk, which we should be avoiding anyway. Perhaps because soy is so abundant, it has become one of the top food allergens people are sensitive to.

As we will see below, soy interferes with the absorption of essential minerals. For example, by reducing selenium absorption, it leads to a reduced ability to make the active form of thyroid hormone. It's as if you're adrift at sea, surrounded by seawater, but one piece is missing from your desalinization kit, so you can't generate drinking water. Your body could be bathed in the primary thyroid hormone T4, but without the ability to convert it to its active form, T3, using selenium, you won't feel the metabolism-boosting effects of your thyroid gland, leaving you tired, mentally slow, and prone to weight gain, with thinning hair, brittle nails, and dry skin.

Soy can also trigger another issue with your thyroid gland. Like lectin-containing foods, soy can lead to autoimmune thyroid disease. Over time, these autoimmune antibodies can destroy enough of the thyroid that you are no longer able to produce enough thyroid hormone for your body to feel energized.

PHYTATES: THE ANTINUTRIENT

Like gluten-containing grains, soy is also rife with phytates, which as discussed earlier are an *antinutrient*. Phytates **interfere** with:

- Absorption of key minerals (especially calcium, copper, magnesium, iron, selenium, and zinc) needed by the body for enzymes to work properly
- Cellular detoxification
- Production of hormones (like testosterone)
- Creation of protective antibodies to viruses and bacteria

As it interferes with calcium and magnesium absorption, soy certainly cannot be good for bone mineral density, especially for post-menopausal women and men older than sixty.

The only way to lessen the effects of this antinutrient is to ferment soy to reduce the phytic acid concentration. Soy, as part of the traditional Asian diet, is consumed in small amounts as fermented miso, tempeh, tofu, and soy sauce, but not to the extent and in all the processed ways we consume it in the West.

If you don't have thyroid or hormonal issues and you lack a sensitivity to soy, you may incorporate small amounts of fermented soy into your diet, but only non–genetically modified (non-GMO), organic soy, and not until *after* the Happy Gut Diet's twenty-eight days of elimination. Like any other food product, the further removed soy is from its natural state through processing, the worse it becomes for us. This brings me to another major issue with soy.

GMO Soy

Greater than 90 percent of the soy mass-produced in the United States is GMO (genetically modified organism). This soy is "Roundup ready"[10] and was the first crop of this type. By genetically modifying a crop to be resistant to an herbicide, farmers can then use an herbicide to kill weeds after the crop has emerged. This is very convenient for farmers but not so convenient for us. The safety and human health effects of GMO crops have never been looked at in a long-term study. Yet as we speak, we are living in one giant population-wide experiment as unlabeled GMO products find their way onto the shelves of local supermarkets disguised in the foods that people frequently consume. For a more detailed discussion of GMOs and why they are bad for us, read *Seeds of Deception* by Jeffrey M. Smith.

For the next twenty-eight days, I want you to say "so long" to soy in your diet. It may be challenging, but I assure you that the benefits outweigh the effort you'll put into changing the way you eat. And with the delicious recipes in Chapter 9, you won't miss the soy.

SCORN THE CORN

Like soy, corn and corn derivatives have infiltrated every corner of our food supply. Cornstarch, corn syrup, dextrose, maltodextrin, and high-fructose corn syrup (HFCS) are a few of the ways that corn products make it into our food and beverages. Although I'll continue to urge you to *read the ingredients,* reading labels won't protect you 100 percent of the time. Corn-fed chickens and cattle predominate in the food industry, so corn may be in your food supply even without your knowledge. You may even be eating eggs from corn-fed chickens. So knowing where your food comes from is critical to becoming a clean eater. With the Happy Gut Diet you will avoid all these types of harmful foods that make it into our daily "nourishment."

Corn itself is a high-glycemic food, meaning that when you eat it your blood sugar will spike in much the same way as consuming cane sugar. It is a sugar equivalent (SE) food. Often, when I ask my patients how much sugar they consume, they answer "not much," but they may actually be consuming sugar in many other less obvious forms. They believe that by not adding sugar to anything or using sugar substitutes, they are avoiding the ravages of sugar on their health. They don't realize that SE foods are just as harmful to us as sugar in terms of what they do to our hormones, like insulin, leading to insulin resistance, leptin resistance, an increased waist circumference, and weight gain. And now with the discovery of two new gluten-like proteins in corn that activate the immune system, we know that corn is a pro-inflammatory food, as are most SE foods. Even more problematic is that most of the corn produced now is GMO.

GMO Corn

As with soy, more than 90 percent of the corn grown in the United States is genetically modified. This GMO corn has also been adapted to be Roundup tolerant and contains residues of this formulation. Another type of GMO corn has been genetically modified to produce Bt toxins, which are used as insecticides. At first glance it seems ingenious to have the corn plant produce its own insect repellant. But think about this for a minute. You could actually be eating corn that produces its own insecticide! What are the potential consequences inside your gut from ingesting Bt toxins? The FDA says it's not significant enough to be toxic, but I beg to differ, and my reasons are in "The Dangers of GMO Corn" on the following page. For the time being, my recommendation is to avoid GMO corn.

Corn is also high in lectins. Lectins bind to the cells lining your intestines, disrupting the tight junctions between the intestinal cells and creating tiny holes that allow larger partially digested food particles to get through. This disrupts your gut flora, leads to inflammation, and eventually causes insulin and leptin resistance. Corn is simply not good for us in the amounts in which it has permeated our food supply.

A sensitivity to corn can result in all sorts of reactions, similar to those from gluten and other food allergens. In my practice, the most common reactions I see are rashes, like eczema (a flaky and occasionally itchy pink skin irritation that occurs in patches and tends to stick around from days to weeks) and hives (itchy, raised red bumps on the skin that can feel hot, can arise within minutes of eating the food, and can cause a great deal of discomfort lasting from minutes to hours). Other food sensitivity issues include migraines, body aches, joint pains, and a depressed mood. Reactions related to its effects as an SE food include fatigue, insomnia, mood swings, hyperactivity in children, sinus congestion, and susceptibility to infections. So avoid this pro-inflammatory food. Scorn the corn! For the twenty-eight-day Elimination Phase of the Happy Gut Diet, you will avoid all corn and corn derivatives.

THE DANGERS OF GMO CORN

Even though there are no double-blind, placebo-controlled human studies, the effects of GMO corn have been studied in laboratory rats, revealing shocking findings. In female rats, hormonal problems prevailed because of the endocrine-disrupting effects of the herbicide (Roundup), and in male rats liver congestion and destruction was the main finding. Both sexes developed very significant kidney problems. Unfortunately, the most detailed tests on GMO safety are only three-month-long feeding trials of laboratory rats. What about their long-term effects on children and adults?

These tests are not independently conducted and are not compulsory for the industry. And when they are conducted, test data and results are often kept secret. What has been most clearly shown in a comparative analysis of the effects of different GMO corn on laboratory rats is that the two organs most affected are the liver and kidneys—the organs of detoxification. Why should ingesting a food that requires immediate detoxification be considered safe for us? Even though we are not lab rats, we cannot ignore the biological effects brought into question. The burden of proof as to the safety of GMOs for human consumption should be on the corporations that produce them, but mandated by food regulatory agencies and carried out by independent, unbiased research institutions. Until this happens and for the time being, my recommendation is to avoid GMO corn.

DON'T PRESUME: AVOID THE LEGUMES (INCLUDING PEANUTS!)

Legumes are plants (or the fruit or seed from such plants) in the family known as *Fabaceae*; they include common foods like alfalfa, beans, carob, chickpeas, lentils, peas, soybeans, tamarind, and peanuts, which are also legumes, not tree nuts. Legumes are high in lectins, as with gluten, soy, and corn. This means legumes pose the same major problems that can lead to inflammation and weight gain as these other foods.

Legumes are also notorious for causing gas, which leads to bloating, abdominal distension, discomfort, and even pain. Anyone who has been doubled over with gas pains knows how bad they can be. Some legumes, such as beans, are worse offenders than others. They contain a type of sugar, an *oligosaccharide* known as a *galactan,* that our digestive tracts cannot break down because we lack the enzyme to do so, but our gut bacteria can, producing hydrogen or methane gas.

Peanuts are another story. Peanuts are a highly allergenic food, and this allergy is often caused by a reaction to peanut proteins. And peanuts are often contaminated with a fungus-produced toxin called *aflatoxin,* which is toxic to humans and provokes strong allergic reactions.

Here are additional reasons to avoid peanuts and products containing them:

- Processed peanut butters often are full of added sugar and sodium to enhance their flavor. This is the sure path to insulin resistance and water retention. Your joints ache, your hands and feet swell, and you can't get rid of that tire around your belly, but you don't realize that what you're eating is causing this.

- Peanuts are full of saturated fats, but not the healthy omega-3 fats found in tree nuts.

- Peanuts, like other legumes, are high in phytates and lectins. They are hard on your digestion, hard on your gut, and hard on your body.

Instead of peanuts and peanut butter, reach for an alternative nut or seed butter, like almond butter which is rich in heart-protective omega-3 fatty acids, and sunflower butter, a source of anti-inflamatory linolenic acid.

A Note on Legumes for Vegans or Vegetarians

If you are vegetarian or vegan, and thus need beans to meet your body's protein demand, there are ways to help make them less problematic, even less gassy, and more comfortable for your digestive system. These steps help lower their phytate content, making them easier to digest and less of an antinutrient for your body. However, remember that legumes have lectins, so it's best to not overdo them.

WAYS TO MAKE YOUR BEANS OR LENTILS LESS GASSY

1. Wash beans or lentils with cold water, then soak lentils for at least 1½ hours and beans overnight in three times the volume of water. After soaking, drain out all the water and then wash the beans again before adding water to cook.
2. Eat beans or lentils alone with no other protein in the same meal.
3. Avoid eating potatoes (remember, they contain lectins) at the same time as beans, as potatoes can interfere with the digestion of beans.
4. Use digestive spices: fennel and ginger added to beans can help make them more digestible.
5. Remember to chew your beans! Savor their flavor, for the digestive process begins in the mouth.
6. Start with easier-to-digest beans, like mung, adzuki, and dal.

FOR SOME, NIGHTSHADES DON'T MAKE THE GRADE

"Nightshade" is the common name used to describe a group of vines, herbs, shrubs, and trees that include well-known members such as mandrake, belladonna, and tobacco. The commonly eaten members of this family include tomatoes, tomatillos, eggplant, potatoes, bell peppers, sweet and hot peppers, pepinos, and pimentos. Although sweet potatoes belong to the same plant order as nightshades, they belong to a different family from the other nightshades here. Nightshades are a particular source of agony for many people who suffer from arthritic conditions or autoimmune disorders. Plants in this family produce alkaloids—a natural insect repellent that can be toxic to humans in large amounts. Common nightshades don't have enough of these alkaloids to be deadly; however, some people with inflammatory conditions are particularly sensitive to even tiny amounts in the diet. In these people, even cooking the nightshades, which will lower the alkaloid content by 40 to 50 percent, will not be enough to save them from the damaging effects.

Like gluten-containing grains, nightshades also harbor lectins or sugar-binding proteins, which can activate the immune system and increase inflammation and pain in the body.

Although removing nightshades is not absolutely required as part of Phase I of the Happy Gut Diet, I strongly recommend that if you have an autoimmune disorder or any arthritic or pain condition, you remove them completely during the twenty-eight-day Elimination Phase. Nightshades may very well be contributing to your pain syndrome, and the only way to know for sure is to remove them for at least four weeks. Then, after this period of elimination, reintroduce them into your diet while observing carefully what symptoms you experience in your body, from several hours up to three days after you consume them. If nightshades are a problem for you, you will be motivated to avoid them by how well you will feel without them.

READY, SET, GO!

Now you see why gluten, eggs, dairy, soy, legumes, corn, and sugar (and, for some of you, nightshades) are inflammatory and are actually making you and your gut sick. Choose the anti-inflammatory foods listed on the shopping list at the end of this chapter instead and follow the Happy Gut Diet program to restore balance to your body. The next chapter will discuss the Gut C.A.R.E. Program in detail, followed by a summary of the daily routine you will follow for the Happy Gut Diet. Use it to help you plan your twenty-eight days to feeling and looking younger and better than ever.

My thirty-four-year-old patient Mark just completed my program, with a few modifications to suit his lifestyle. When he came to see me, he was overweight with an elevated waist circumference, which put him at high risk for diabetes, heart disease, and stroke. In fact, his blood tests were already showing signs of metabolic syndrome, a precursor to diabetes. However, in just twenty-eight days, he underwent a remarkable transformation. As a result, he has used it as the springboard to a healthier way of living. I hope Mark's story inspires you to make these changes and come out feeling better and stronger. This is what Mark has to say:

> *Changing my eating habits has been the hardest thing I've ever done. I wasn't being mindful about what I was eating, or how I was eating. Like so many others, I was addicted to the salt, sugar, and fat in processed "foods," as well as caffeine to keep me going since I wasn't getting proper energy or nourishment. Every day I would skip breakfast and lunch, then overdo it on pasta and bread or takeout for dinner, pass out, and repeat the cycle.*
>
> *As Dr. Pedre explained, I needed to make my health a top priority and make the choice every day to focus on what was best in the long term. He suggested I give up wheat (bread, pasta), dairy, soy, and coffee.*

Even though I knew it was for the best, I almost gave up on the first day—my body wanted what it was used to. I had a terrible headache that night and wasn't sure if I could break these addictions. But I didn't cave, and it's gotten easier every day after that. Instead of coffee, I drink green tea. I'm grilling chicken and fish instead of eating fried foods. I'm drinking fruit/vegetable smoothies instead of milk, and I no longer eat a pint of ice cream a night. After twenty-eight days, I've lost eleven pounds and an inch and a quarter off my waist, and I am sleeping better, but most gratifying of all is finally breaking those habits and knowing I'm stronger than the addictions.

THE HAPPY GUT SHOPPING LIST

To prep your pantry for the twenty-eight-day Happy Gut Diet and make it easier for you to find the foods you can have when you shop, here is a more comprehensive list of which foods are in and which foods are generally out in the Happy Gut Diet.

WHAT'S IN	WHAT'S OUT
Vegetables	
All leafy greens	White potatoes, yams, corn
Whole vegetables (raw, steamed, baked, sautéed, juiced, or roasted)	If excessive gassiness, avoid onions, garlic, cabbage, and Brussels sprouts
Sweet potatoes, beets, pumpkin, butternut or spaghetti squash	Nightshades[11] (tomatoes, eggplant, peppers, red goji berries, etc.) and legumes (beans and lentils, except peas and chickpeas)
Garbanzo beans (chickpeas), peas, and sea vegetables	
Limited amount of onions and garlic	
Fruit	
Fresh or frozen berries	Fruit juices
Organic green apples, oranges, lemons, and limes	All other fruits, including red apples and dried fruits (except in very limited amounts)

WHAT'S IN	WHAT'S OUT
Dairy Substitutes/Dairy	
Organic, grass-fed ghee[12]	Milk, cream, butter, cheese, cottage cheese, yogurt, nondairy creamer, ice cream
Hemp and nut milks (almond,[13] hazelnut, cashew, etc.)	Dairy proteins (casein, whey)
Coconut milk and coconut oil	Milk chocolate
	Eggs and egg substitutes
Grains	
Quinoa, millet, amaranth, buckwheat, brown rice, rice bran, gluten-free oats (preferably steel-cut), and teff	Wheat, gluten-containing grains (fu, farro, durum, barley, rye, malt, orzo, bulgur, oats, couscous, spelt, semolina, seitan, and triticale)
Meat and Fish	
Lean, grass-fed beef	Corn- or grain-fed, factory-farmed meats
Lamb	Cold cuts, cured meats, canned meats, hot dogs
Duck	Farm-raised fish
Free-range, hormone- and antibiotic-free chicken and turkey	
Wild game (rabbit, bison, venison, elk, pheasant, etc.)	
Fresh or flash-frozen wild cold-water fish (salmon, sockeye salmon, halibut, sardines, low-mercury tuna, etc.)	
Nuts and Seeds	
Almonds, walnuts, hemp, sesame, sunflower seeds, pistachios, Brazil nuts, macadamia nuts	Peanuts and peanut butter
Nut and seed butters (almond, sesame, sunflower, etc.)	
Limited amounts of cashews and pecans	
Vegetable Proteins	
Bee pollen, spirulina, and blue-green algae (chlorella)	Beans, soybeans (including soy sauce and soybean oil)

WHAT'S IN	WHAT'S OUT
Fats and Oils	
Extra-virgin olive, coconut, avocado, safflower, sunflower, sesame, flax, almond, and walnut oils	Hydrogenated oils, canola oil, and any processed oils
Coconut and avocado	Mayonnaise
Organic ghee from grassfed cows	Margarine, butter, shortening
Drinks	
Filtered, reverse-osmosis, alkaline water[14] and limited amounts of mineral waters	Alcohol
Green, white, jasmine, oolong, and herbal teas; yerba maté	Coffee, caffeinated beverages (except for teas, like green)
Limited amounts of coconut water	Sodas, bottled teas (tend to be loaded with sugar), and fruit juices (even those with heart-healthy labels, like pomegranate, are full of sugar)
Juiced green vegetables	
Sweeteners	
Limited amounts of stevia, xylitol,[15] erythritol	White and brown sugar, refined sugar, high-fructose corn syrup, brown rice syrup
Very limited amounts of the following: honey, maple syrup, organic dried cane syrup, and coconut sugar	Evaporated cane juice, artificial sweeteners (aspartame, sucralose, acesulfame potassium, Sweet'N Low, Equal, and Splenda), juice concentrates, and agave nectar
Condiments	
All herbs/spices, sea salt, black pepper	Sauces (barbecue, teriyaki, soy, etc.)
Carob; raw, dairy-free, sugar-free chocolate	Vinegars (except apple cider or limited quantities of other types)
Stone-ground mustard	Commercial salad dressings
Gluten-free tamari	Ketchup
Coconut aminos	Relish, chutney
Bragg Liquid Aminos and Bragg Organic Apple Cider Vinegar, other vinegars (only in limited quantities)	
Fennel seeds (as a digestive and breath freshener)	

PART II

THE GUT C.A.R.E. PROGRAM:

TWENTY-EIGHT DAYS TO A NEW YOU

ELIMINATE SYMPTOMS AND MAINTAIN YOUR HEALTH WITH THE GUT C.A.R.E. PROGRAM

N OW THAT YOU KNOW why your gut is unhappy, you're ready to get started repairing it, optimizing your health, and improving how you feel on a daily basis. Like many of the patients who come see me on a weekly basis, you are tired of feeling exhausted, bloated, crampy, gassy, achy, and pained, and you're ready to make the changes that will clear up your health issues for good. All I ask of you is a commitment—give the Gut C.A.R.E. Program twenty-eight days to transform your health!

Once again, a reminder of what C.A.R.E. stands for:

CLEANSE	Remove gut irritants, infections, food sensitivities, and toxins in food
ACTIVATE	Reactivate healthy digestion by replacing essential nutrients and enzymes
RESTORE	Reintroduce beneficial bacteria for a healthy gut flora
ENHANCE	Repair, regenerate, and heal the intestinal lining

For a seamless Gut C.A.R.E. journey, in this chapter you will find an overview of how to implement each of the four program steps. As part of the Gut C.A.R.E. Program, I developed a series of complementary supplements to fast-track you along the path to wellness. For the morning breakfast smoothies, you'll find a gut-healing, fructose-free, hypoallergenic, vegan protein powder designed to support your gut health and promote balanced detoxification. In addition, I carefully selected a series of easy-to-swallow encapsulated supplements to support digestive wellness, along with a high-potency probiotic to promote healthy gut microflora. This line of supplements can be found at www.happygutlife.com, but you may also complete the program by using the supplement checklist at the end of this chapter to guide you on what to purchase.

To make it even easier, I have also provided a detailed template to guide you through each day—A Day on the Happy Gut Diet (page 109)—including when to take the supplements. If you need more support, visit the Happy Gut Life website, where you will find more educational resources and recipes and have the ability to connect with a Happy Gut–Certified Health Coach who can help steer you through the program.

C.A.R.E.: YOUR GUT REBOOT SYSTEM

C.A.R.E., in all senses of the word, is a *gut reboot system*. It is how you are going to restore and repair the normal activity of your gut. It will help reestablish balance in an imbalanced system. By fixing your gut—your primary organ for assimilation of nutrients and barrier to the outside world—you will feel the benefits throughout your entire body.

Why Twenty-Eight Days?

If you've been eating a diet that is making you and your gut sick, it takes a minimum of two weeks for your body to begin to heal from all the inflammatory foods you were eating. That means that it can take two weeks for you to start to feel the positive effects of the dietary changes that are part of the Gut C.A.R.E. Program. For some the changes are noticeable within a few days, but for others it may take longer than two weeks. It depends on how sick you were at the start of the program.

Begin by taking four days while reading *Happy Gut* to fill out the pre-program food journal (in Appendix A) so you can see how you are currently eating, whether consciously or unconsciously. Once that's done, fill out the Happy Gut Pre-Program Symptoms Questionnaire at the beginning of the twenty-eight days so you can see for yourself how your symptoms shift at the end (you'll find the Pre-Program SQ at the end of Chapter 1 and the Post-Program SQ in Appendix B).

No matter what challenges you face, the Gut C.A.R.E. Program is designed to assist your body so you can lose the bloat, drop the weight, feel and look younger, and be mentally clearer. During the first week, you may actually not feel so great. As your body detoxes from the foods on the "Out" list (see pages 71–73), you may go through a healing crisis. These foods, food additives, or sweeteners are either the most difficult for our bodies to break down or are the most likely to bog down your liver as it works to detoxify them.

The last two weeks of the twenty-eight-day Gut C.A.R.E. Program are your gut-stabilizing phase; this is when the healing really takes place. Your body has cleared the food antigen-antibody complexes that were bogging down your immune system, and the cells that line your intestines (called *enterocytes*) are beginning to mend. Tight junctions between the cells are reinforced, and the leakiness or hyperpermeability of your gut is improving. Food particles are digesting better with the Gut C.A.R.E. Program supplements, and weight loss continues as your internal inflammation and leaky gut heal.

Twenty-eight days—it's all I ask for. I can tell you from having worked with all sorts of people that even the ones who thought they could not do this managed to do it successfully. You can do it as well!

Gut C.A.R.E. and Care of the Self

In our modern, fast-paced world, the care of the self has been lost. Our lives are spent rushing to the next appointment or next client meeting, or "chained" to our desks in a nine-to-five job that actually ends up being nine-to-seven or later. We are often eating on the run or at our desks, or skipping meals because we don't have time. If you are required to sit all day, your order-in options are often not the greatest, and without applying mindfulness, your eating becomes something that is inserted into the other activities in your life rather than the moment of peace, reflection, and transcendence that it should be.

C.A.R.E. is first about consciousness. It is about *self-care*. It is about kindness to the self in the way we prepare or acquire our food, the way we eat, and the company in which we eat. Eating should be a ritual in our daily lives.

The expression "stop and smell the roses" should really be "stop and smell your food." Take in the aromas, slow down, chew your food carefully, don't gulp it down. Breathe, open up your chest, don't cross your arms. Engage in conversation, think happy thoughts, be thankful. Share, enjoy the flavors, and savor each part of your meal.

Sure, C.A.R.E. is also an acronym for the steps I am about to explain, but the word "care" was chosen to express so much more than just those steps. It is the way I want you to think about what you are doing as you embark on the Gut C.A.R.E. Program. Eating was a ritual in the cultures of old, and even today it should still be an event, not just something that is stuck in between tasks so you can keep moving in your hectic life.

Care for yourself. Care for each other and make it a family affair. Love is often expressed through food, so let the way you choose to eat be an expression of love for yourself. Think about how you've been eating. Go back to the four-day pre-program food journal (see Appendix A), and think about where you were not kind to yourself. Where did you make choices out of stress or impulsiveness, or because you waited too long to eat so you were starving? Ask yourself how you can love yourself better through the C.A.R.E. of what you choose to eat, how you eat, and when you eat. Make food something that nourishes you at all levels—body, mind, and spirit.

CLEANSE

Cleanse ⇨ Eliminate harmful substances and organisms (such as parasites, yeast, or unfriendly bacteria) and the foods we discussed in Chapter 2 that contribute to poor gut health. Replace harmful thoughts with gratitude.

In the simplest terms, to cleanse is to clear out everything that is impure or bad from your body. The problem is that to cleanse can mean different things to different people. Are you abstaining from sugar and sweets? You might abstain from alcohol for one month. But what about all the other things you may be consuming that are just as toxic and taxing to your body?

ELIMINATE HIGH-SENSITIVITY FOODS

Identifying and eliminating the foods and environmental toxins that rob your body of energy are at the heart of the first step of the Gut C.A.R.E. Program.

Over the course of a lifetime, the average adult will consume between thirty and sixty tons of food. So even though when cleansing you want to eliminate the unseen pathogens in your gut—bacteria, viruses, yeast, parasites, and environmental toxic substances—the worst offenders are often the artificial substances, fillers, food dyes, processed foods, and sweeteners you eat on a daily basis that are causing a toxic buildup in your body and must be eliminated. The foods you eat not only determine the state of your internal bacterial environment, but they pose a huge load of antigenic substances that can activate your gut-associated immune system.

The best way to cleanse the body is to remove the most common food allergens, intolerances, and sensitivities from the diet. You will also avoid alcohol and coffee. Some foods that may be considered part of a healthy diet have been omitted from this program; in the interest of a happy gut, they are temporarily left out to allow gut healing to take place. Don't worry, once you've completed the twenty-eight days, I will help you reintroduce the foods back into your diet.

Here's a reminder of the macro-principles of the Happy Gut Diet; a more detailed shopping list is in Chapter 2 on pages 71–73:

WHAT'S IN	WHAT'S OUT
Fresh vegetables	Wheat/gluten
Dark, leafy greens	Lentils, beans
Quinoa	White rice
Brown rice	White potatoes
Sweet potatoes	Dairy/butter
Ghee (clarified butter)	Coffee
Green and/or herbal teas	Alcohol
Fermented foods (kimchi, sauerkraut)	Processed or artificial sugar
Nuts, seeds, and nut butters	Corn
Avocado	Hydrogenated oils, trans fats
Coconut, coconut oil	Almost all fruits
Fresh or frozen berries	Farm-raised fish
Wild fish	Grain-raised meats
Free-range, antibiotic-free poultry	Nonorganic Eggs
Grass-fed meats	
Wild game	
Organic, free-range eggs*	

*Eggs are allowed as a reintroduction food after the twenty-eight days.

HAPPY GUT PRINCIPLES

The Happy Gut Diet focuses on clean ingredients with foods that are easy to digest, low in fructose and sugar, and devoid of the substances that are hard on the gut. The emphasis is on foods that are organic, pesticide-free, non-GMO, full of healthy fats, locally grown, and sustainably farmed. And when I say locally grown, I mean support your local farmers. Become part of a CSA (community-supported agriculture).

WHAT TO EAT

1. Organic (non-GMO)
2. Healthy fats
3. Nuts/seeds
4. High-fiber, low-glycemic carbs
5. Nonstarchy vegetables
6. Hypoallergenic proteins (peas, rice, chia, and hemp)
7. Clean and lean proteins:
   - Hormone-free, pasture-raised beef, lamb
   - Free-range chicken and turkey
   - Wild-caught cold-water fish (no farmed fish)
   - Wild game

With these principles, you don't need to count calories! When you give the body the right nutrition, you won't need to fill it with endless calories from low-nutrient, calorie-dense foods that leave it wanting more and more but never sate its true needs. You will feel energized by the richness of a power-packed, phytonutrient-dense way of eating. For these reasons, I want you to use the twenty-eight days as a kickoff to changes that you can incorporate into a new philosophy of living and eating.

By avoiding gluten/wheat, dairy, soy, corn, legumes, and added sugar, you will be following what is known as an *oligoantigenic diet* (meaning a diet that is low in foods that are known to cause immune responses or lead to intolerances).[1] Those of you with autoimmune conditions, arthritis, or body aches and pains will also avoid the nightshades.

In addition to food allergies, sensitivities, and intolerances, there are other contaminants in the foods we eat and the water we drink that we need to be aware of for the "cleanse" portion of the Gut C.A.R.E. Program.

DRINK CLEAN WATER

Pharmaceutical residues have been found in the watersheds of twenty-four metropolitan areas in the United States, and these affect the drinking water supplies of approximately 41 million Americans, possibly more. This means drug metabolites—such as from antibiotics, anticonvulsants, mood stabilizers, and sex hormones—have been found in these drinking water supplies. Not even the pristine lakes in the Swiss Alps have been left untouched! Think about that before you fill up a glass of water from the tap.

Drug metabolites are not the only problem. Our drinking water is heavily chlorinated to keep it free of bacteria, viruses, and parasites. Unfortunately, ingesting chlorine is not ideal for optimal health, as it can interfere with the functioning of the thyroid gland—the master of our metabolism. In addition, heavy metals have found their way into drinking water supplies. One recent study found late-term miscarriages and spontaneous abortions, linked to drinking water, occurred at an unusually high rate among women in Washington, D.C. During the same time period, lead levels were dangerously high in Washington's drinking water because of lead pipes.[2] So whether it's chlorine, fluoride, or heavy metals in your water, or drug metabolites that were not removed by a water treatment plant, the water that comes from the tap is far from clean and clear of toxins. It is not friendly to your gut.

As part of the Cleanse portion of the Gut C.A.R.E. Program, here are my recommendations for improving your drinking water:

1. **Carbon filters** remove chlorine and fluoride in water, giving it a cleaner taste. This is the simplest to implement and can be purchased as an easy-to-use standalone water filter such as a Brita, PUR, Aquasana, or ZeroWater.

2. **Distilled water** can be purchased in plastic containers, but beware of BPA (bisphenol-A, an endocrine disruptor derived from petroleum that mimics estrogen in the body and can cause hormonal abnormalities that are not easily detectable through laboratory tests) and other toxins in plastic. Drinking distilled water may benefit someone undergoing a heavy metal detox, but not without properly replenishing trace and essential minerals. This choice should only be made under the supervision of a physician or health-care practitioner skilled in detoxification.

3. **Reverse osmosis systems** remove drug metabolites, heavy metal ions, and chlorine from tap water. This type of in-home water treatment system usually requires a professional installation, although there are do-it-yourself kits you can purchase at stores such as Home Depot.

4. **Electrolyzed reduced (ER) or electrolyzed oxidized (EO) water**—the normal pH of tap water is 6.5 to 8.5, but water has an alkaline pH when electrolyzed reduced, or an acidic pH when oxidized. Studies have shown the benefits of these types of water for a variety of reasons. ER water (pH 11.6) and EO water (pH 2.3) were found in one study to reduce pesticide residues on vegetables significantly better than tap water or detergent, without affecting the nutrient content of the vegetables.[3] This is an excellent way to make nonorganic produce safer for consumption.

The sicker you are, the more you should consider that investing in one of these systems is ultimately an investment in your health and the health of your family. However, if you are on a budget, start with an activated carbon filter, such as the Brita, PUR, or Aquasana.

A GREENER KITCHEN MEANS A HEALTHIER YOU

Everyday items used in food storage, cookware, and cooking utensils often harbor engineered compounds that pose potent, silent health threats to our bodies. Many of these compounds bioaccumulate over years and are stored in the fat of the body. In a study done by the Environmental Working Group, 287 industrial chemicals were found in the umbilical cord blood from ten newborns. "Among them are eight perfluorochemicals used as stain and oil repellants in fast food packaging, clothes and textiles—including the Teflon chemical PFOA, recently characterized as a likely human carcinogen by the EPA's Science Advisory Board . . ."[4]

The brands mentioned below are used as examples, and by no means do they represent all the "green" brands that can replace your common kitchen items. I want to help you be an educated consumer. Read labels and research the products you use on a daily basis. I use many of these items in my own kitchen.

Cookware

Nonstick pans and cooking utensils are convenient, but at what price? PFOA (perfluorooctanoic acid), an ingredient in nonstick surfaces such as Teflon, has been implicated as a causative environmental toxin in autism spectrum disorders.[5] Persistent organic pollutants (POPs) enter our bodies when we eat the foods we prepare on these surfaces, and then they have no easy way out. That is why they are called "persistent." They stay in your body for a literal eternity, pocketed wherever fat is stored in the body. In fact, over time these POPs slowly poison your cellular energy machinery, making you gain weight and feel tired and leaving you prone to diseases that are not easily traced back to an exposure. Organic pollutants have even been implicated in the worldwide explosion of the rates of diabetes and obesity.[6]

"Cleanse" your kitchen by looking for cookware labeled "PFOA-free" and "PTFE-free" and avoiding PFOA and PTFE (polytetrafluoroethylene) in nonstick surfaces.

POTS AND PANS FOR GREEN COOKING

1. Ceramic-coated nonstick, such as Bialetti's Aeternum collection
2. Porcelain-enameled cast iron, such as Le Creuset
3. Stainless steel (great for making rice and soups and steaming vegetables)

For example, 360 Cookware's stainless steel products with Vapor technology offer a healthier alternative to cooking with oils. With my 360 Cookware sauté pan, I make perfectly steamed broccoli in less than five minutes, using very little water, thus retaining all the nutritional value of the food. See Appendix D for a special 360 Cookware offer. Who said preparing a healthy, gut-friendly meal had to take a long time?

Don't forget that your utensils are often manufactured with nonstick surfaces as well, which can be toxic to you. Instead, use utensils made from:

- Bamboo (a renewable, nontoxic resource)
- Stainless steel

Food Storage

We all appreciate the convenience, environmental consciousness, and anti-wasting influence of food storage containers. However, avoid plastic food storage containers, which contain BPA or other bisphenols. Instead, use containers made from glass or Pyrex.

Plastic wrap:

Avoid plastic wraps that use polyvinylidene chloride (such as Saran) and choose a wrap that is made from polyethylene (less evil). An example of the less toxic version is Glad ClingWrap. Even better yet, forgo the plastic wrap and instead use old-fashioned wax paper with tape to hold it together if necessary.

Dishwashing Soap

Avoid triclosan, an antibacterial agent, and just use regular plant-based detergent, such as Seventh Generation Natural Dish Liquid. You don't need an antibacterial agent unless you are planning on sterilizing your apartment like a hospital.

DANGERS OF MICROWAVE OVENS

Avoid heating food in microwaves because it may reduce the nutrient value of the food.

Microwave ovens often leak microwaves through the door. These are one form of electromagnetic forces (EMFs) that will make some people feel fatigued and even depressed.

- Never microwave food in plastic containers, because the BPA, an endocrine hormone disruptor, in the plastic will leach into the food you are about to ingest.
- Microwave popcorn is probably the worst and most toxic because of the fire-retardant materials in the lining of the bag.
- Try to avoid reheating food in a microwave oven whenever possible.
- If you do own a microwave oven (no judgments), never stand in front of it while it is on. Use it as little as possible, and try to use a toaster oven instead. It really takes only a couple of minutes extra to heat up leftovers on the stovetop or in an oven.

CLEANSE YOUR MIND

If you are cleansing your gut of all the detrimental foods and substances you expose it to and ridding it of the bacteria, viruses, or parasites that are harmful to you, you cannot neglect cleansing your mind. During these twenty-eight days, take time to express positive feelings of well-being. Purge your mind of destructive thoughts—that inner voice that says, "No matter what I do, I will continue to feel sick, so I might as well eat the things I crave regardless of how they make me feel." By the end of the first week on the Happy Gut Diet, your mind will stop craving the foods that are bad for you.

Start with Gratitude

In your food journal (see Appendix B), start your day by writing what you are grateful for. It can be the simplest thing. Gratitude engenders positive thoughts and is a great way to get out of negative thinking patterns. No matter how bad you feel, there is always something to be grateful for. Get into the practice of expressing a *daily gratitude,* and you will see that your life will change. For the next twenty-eight days, write down a daily gratitude in your food journal, embrace the changes you are making, and say good-bye to the naysayer in your head. Look to where you are fortunate in your life.

At the end of the twenty-eight days, take your long list of gratitudes and put them together on a piece of paper, or poster board, or type them out. Be creative. Make a vision board with your gratitudes and add pictures of how you see yourself in wellness and/or things you want to do when you are at your best health. This will help keep you motivated once you are done with the program and are moving on to a plan for life.

HOW TO IMPLEMENT CLEANSE DAILY

1. Eliminate all high-sensitivity foods listed in Chapter 2, along with coffee and alcohol.

2. Take the Gut C.A.R.E. CLEANSE supplement (summarized at the end of the chapter) three times daily before meals.
3. Prepare the Gut C.A.R.E. CLEANSE SHAKE using one of the seven breakfast smoothie recipes in Chapter 9.
4. Drink clean water.
5. Create a greener kitchen.
6. Cleanse your mind.
7. Express a daily gratitude. Record this in your food/symptom journal in Appendix B.

ACTIVATE

Activate ⇨ Reactivate the healthy function of the gut by bridging any gaps or deficiencies in the digestive process using supplements that replenish digestive enzymes, bile salts, stomach acids, minerals, vitamins, hypoallergenic proteins, healthy fats, and fiber.

An imbalanced gut will not produce the enzymes it needs in sufficient quantities to break down foods, resulting in many of the uncomfortable gut and body symptoms you may be feeling.

The main enzymes that may require replacement are:

- **Amylases**—digest carbohydrates into single sugars (mainly glucose)
- **Proteases**—digest proteins to usable amino acids
- **Lipases**—break down fats
- **Bile salts**—emulsify fats, remove cholesterol and toxins (drugs, heavy metals)

Other enzymes that may require replacement include:

- **Cellulases**—break down plant cell walls
- **Saccharidases**—break down simple sugars

These are normally secreted by the cells of the intestinal lining or by the liver, gallbladder, and pancreas into the gut lumen. But when the gut is inflamed, these cells and organs begin to malfunction.

Other components of digestion that may be deficient and require replacement through supplementation are hydrochloric acid (produced in the stomach) and bile (synthesized by your liver).

LOW STOMACH ACID (HYPOCHLORHYDRIA)

As we age, our stomach acid production drops, and even though you may have symptoms of hyperacidity, you may actually not be producing enough stomach acid. The most commonly acquired causes of low stomach acid are the over-the-counter (OTC) medications known as H_2 blockers and proton pump inhibitors (PPIs).

Common causes of low stomach acid (hypochlorhydria) include:

• Aging
• Stress
• Fasting
• Chronic viral or bacterial infections
• Any debilitating chronic condition
• PPIs (for example, Aciphex, Nexium, Prilosec, Protonix)
• H_2 blockers (for example, Zantac, Ranitidine, Tagamet)
• Overconsumption of antacids (for example, Tums, Rolaids)

Low stomach acid often leads to:

• SIBO (small intestine bacterial overgrowth, discussed in Chapter 6)
• Yeast overgrowth
• Calcium malabsorption (which may lead to osteoporosis)

- An increased risk of bacterial infections[7]
- An inability to efficiently break down protein, which can even result in depression because of a deficiency of the amino acids needed to create neurotransmitters for healthy brain function

---

THE TRUTH ABOUT ACID-BLOCKING MEDICATIONS

The number of people in the United States who take acid blockers (H_2 blockers and PPIs) on a daily basis is estimated at more than 100 million; worldwide, acid-blocking medications (like Nexium and Prilosec) have become among the most widely prescribed class of drugs. In one study, hospitalized patients given an acid-blocking medication were found to have a 74 percent increased risk of acquiring a *Clostridium difficile* infection, a hard-to-treat bacterial intestinal infection that may occur in people who have been treated with antibiotics. Stomach acid is there to protect against this bacteria and others.

If you are older than sixty, you are also more likely to have low stomach acid, resulting in digestive problems. Other nutrients that may become deficient as a result of low stomach acid or acid-blocking medications include vitamins B_6, B_{12}, folic acid, and iron. And since the production of stomach acid is zinc dependent, having low stomach acid could be caused by a zinc deficiency.[8]

WHY USE DIGESTIVE ENZYME SUPPLEMENTS?

By "activating" digestion through digestive enzyme supplementation, we improve the breakdown of proteins, fats, and carbohydrates, and if you can break down your food into its component parts, you stop reacting (because our bodies don't react to broken-down molecules, such as amino acids).

Protease enzymes act as a catalyst to break down protein into amino acids. They can even help split up partially digested dietary proteins that entered through the leaky gut, as well as break apart food antigen-immune complexes that are already in the circulation and that tend to deposit in your joints, where they lead to pain from inflammation. Digestive enzymes, like Wobenzym, taken on an empty stomach between meals can reduce this inflammation and pain.

"Activate" is a key step in healing your gut and improving your nutrient absorption. Once we have activated your digestive processes, we are ready for the next step. It's time to Restore what is missing in your gut ecosystem.

HOW TO IMPLEMENT ACTIVATE DAILY

1. Start with the Gut C.A.R.E. Program ACTIVATE digestive enzyme support three times daily, fifteen minutes before each meal of the day.
2. Add a betaine HCl (acid supplement) of 650 milligrams with protein-rich meals if you have signs and symptoms of low stomach acid. (See Chapter 6 for an easy-to-do home test to assess whether you are suffering from low stomach acid production.)
3. Start each day with a Happy Gut breakfast smoothie (see Chapter 9), which contains raw, enzyme-rich foods.
4. Work with a Functional Medicine practitioner to figure out any specific areas, such as fat digestion and absorption or protein malabsorption, where you may need extra support.
5. Take the Gut C.A.R.E. RELAX supplement (two capsules) or the recommended remedies for bowel regularity (see page 114) before heading to bed each night if you tend toward constipation.

Restore ⇨ Use probiotics and prebiotics to reinoculate the intestines with friendly flora (microorganisms that are beneficial to health) and promote their proliferation.

The third step in the Gut C.A.R.E. Program is meant to reestablish microbial balance in your gut ecosystem. We want to reintroduce the favorable bacteria, or probiotics, that were decimated by all types of gut insults, most notably antibiotics, unfavorable bacterial infections, parasites, and yeast.

BEGIN TO RESTORE WITH PROBIOTICS

It doesn't matter if you've taken antibiotics only once every year or only a few times in your life. Each instance you have been on antibiotics, your gut flora is disrupted. We're talking about more than five hundred different species of microorganisms residing in the human gut and totaling in the trillions (that's more than the number of cells in our bodies and even the number of stars in the Milky Way!), whose delicate balance not only influences gut function but also our overall health. A disruption in our gut flora then opens the door for unfriendly microbes to step in and take over.

Why Are Probiotics So Important?

A vital component of the gut ecosystem are the favorable probiotic bacteria that help us maintain proper intestinal permeability. They serve various purposes, but one of their most important functions is their ability to outnumber and antagonize unwelcome pathogens in the GI tract. These pathogens could be other unfavorable bacteria, yeast, or parasites. This ability is called "colonization resistance"—in other words, they prevent the colonization of our guts by unfavorable pathogens. Studies have indicated that our normal flora even secretes its own antimicrobials.[9]

Probiotics—our little helpers—also compete against unfavorable flora for bacterial binding sites on the inside lining of our intestines, which is yet another mechanism by which they protect us from harmful pathogens.

PROBIOTICS HELP IMPROVE GUT IMMUNITY

Oral administration of a probiotic called *L. casei GG* has been shown to increase gut immunity in patients with Crohn's disease by stimulating the release of secretory immunoglobulin A (SIgA), a protective antibody that our immune systems secrete throughout our mucosal surfaces (meaning the linings of both our airways and gut) as a first line of defense against microbes.[10]

Probiotics not only protect against pathogens by inhibiting or neutralizing their activity, they also help reduce the "leakiness" of the gut and bolster our immune system in ways that help protect us. Probiotic supplements have many other positive benefits as well; for example, they have been shown to decrease the frequency of sinus, ear, and upper respiratory infections in susceptible children.[11,12]

CULTURED FOODS, PROBIOTIC BOOSTERS

Of note for those with lactose intolerance: certain cultured dairy products may not be as hard on the digestive system because of the fermentation (partial breakdown of the lactose sugar) that occurs in its production. A number of fermented and cultured foods can support the growth and proliferation of your "good" bacteria. You'll want to incorporate some of these:

- Cultured foods, such as yogurts or kefir[13]
- Fermented foods, such as fermented vegetables, sauerkraut, and kimchi
- Cultured beverages containing favorable live bacteria, such as kombucha or Coconut Water Kefir (see recipe in Chapter 9)

However, when starting the Gut C.A.R.E. Program, it is best to avoid all dairy for twenty-eight days, then, when reintroducing, start with organic, rBGH-free, cultured dairy products.

You can also take a probiotic supplement containing freeze-dried bacteria in a powder, tablet, or capsule; see Appendix C for brands that are lactose-free and dairy-free. Normally, probiotics require refrigeration and come with an expiration date, after which the potency on the bottle can no longer be guaranteed. The dose of a probiotic may range from 5 billion CFUs (an acronym for "colony-forming units," the measure used to express its potency) to 30, 50, or even 100 billion CFUs. The sicker your gut is—in other words, the more imbalanced it is—the higher the probiotic dose that will be required to create a positive effect. It is safe to start at 30 to 50 billion CFUs, but you should work with a health practitioner to guide you on any dose changes.

Although there are endless species of beneficial bacteria that could be discussed, I am going to focus on the two most commonly used in supplements.

Lactobacillus *and* Bifidobacterium:

Lactobacillus predominantly live in the small bowel (the portion of the gut that follows the stomach). Probiotics containing *Lactobacillus sp.* help to repopulate the small intestine with friendly organisms that will help support digestion and the performance of the immune system. The most beneficial are *L. acidophilus*, *L. plantarum*, and *L. paracasei*.

The *Bifidobacteria* (*Bifidus*) predominantly live in the colon or large intestine. They produce butyrate, which is essential for the health of the cells that line the colon, supplying their energy needs so they can function optimally. This is a very important symbiotic relationship. The most beneficial of these are *B. lactis* and *B. longum*. Studies have shown that *B. lactis* helps support normal intestinal motility, promotes immune balance, and relieves IBS-like symptoms.

How to take probiotics:

- Look for dairy-free probiotics that contain at least 15 billion CFUs each of *Lactobacillus* and *Bifidobacterium* (a total of 30 billion CFUs) guaranteed by the manufacturer through the expiration date.
- Take on an empty stomach twice a day for at least three months.
- Keep the probiotics refrigerated after opening to maintain their freshness and potency longer.
- If you have a leaky gut or inflammatory bowel disease (such as Crohn's or ulcerative colitis), you may need to take up to a total of 200 billion CFUs daily.
- For suggestions on quality probiotic supplements, see Appendix C.

Probiotics for Inflammatory Bowel Diseases

For patients with inflammatory bowel disease, such as ulcerative colitis or Crohn's disease, double-blind placebo-controlled trials have shown the benefits of probiotic microorganisms in preventing recurrences and reducing symptoms. One product (VSL#3) containing a combination of favorable strains has been shown to be as effective as standard therapy in preventing relapses in chronic pouchitis, ulcerative colitis, and Crohn's disease.[14,15]

BENEFITS OF
PROBIOTICS & PREBIOTICS

Mutually beneficial effects of probiotic bacteria and
their food substrates in human hosts.

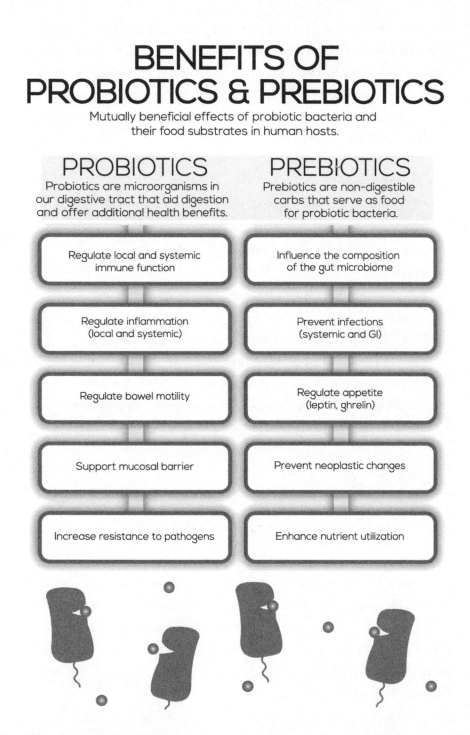

PROBIOTICS

Probiotics are microorganisms in
our digestive tract that aid digestion
and offer additional health benefits.

PREBIOTICS

Prebiotics are non-digestible
carbs that serve as food
for probiotic bacteria.

PROBIOTICS	PREBIOTICS
Regulate local and systemic immune function	Influence the composition of the gut microbiome
Regulate inflammation (local and systemic)	Prevent infections (systemic and GI)
Regulate bowel motility	Regulate appetite (leptin, ghrelin)
Support mucosal barrier	Prevent neoplastic changes
Increase resistance to pathogens	Enhance nutrient utilization

PREBIOTICS: IT'S ALL ABOUT FIBER

Prebiotics are nondigestible fibers found in foods such as Jerusalem artichokes and raw scallions. Part of the Restore step of the Gut C.A.R.E. Program involves "feeding" the healthy microflora with prebiotics. These compounds promote the growth of beneficial flora.

THE TOP FOODS CONTAINING PREBIOTICS

1. Raw chicory root: prebiotic content is about 65 percent of chicory root's total weight
2. Raw Jerusalem artichoke: 32 percent of total weight
3. Raw dandelion greens: 24 percent of total weight (also great for liver and kidney detoxification)
4. Raw garlic: 18 percent of total weight
5. Raw leeks: 12 percent of total weight
6. Raw onions (including scallions): 9 percent of total weight
7. Cooked onion: 5 percent of total weight
8. Asparagus: 5 percent of total weight
9. Raw banana: 1 percent of total weight

How to take prebiotics:

The best way to get your prebiotics is to eat them. Incorporate more foods rich in prebiotics into your diet, but do so slowly. Going too fast in increasing your prebiotic foods can make you gassier. You may also take prebiotics in a supplement, but it is best to do this under the supervision of a health-care professional.

Soluble Fibers for Digestion Modulation

Soluble fibers are important because they help you feel full by attracting water and forming a gel-like substance during digestion. This delays the emptying of your stomach. They also slow the rate at which the sugars that are broken down from carbohydrates enter the bloodstream, helping to blunt the insulin response. This in turn reduces the harmful effects insulin has in the body—namely weight gain and the accumulation of belly fat, especially the dangerous fat around the internal organs. Soluble fibers also interfere with the absorption of cholesterol, thus helping to lower LDL ("bad") cholesterol. Soluble fibers also function as a prebiotic for our favorable gut flora.

Thus, soluble fibers are an important part of a gut-healthy diet. During the Happy Gut Diet, start with the allowed foods, then incorporate more foods rich in soluble fibers after the twenty-eight days.

These are among the best sources of soluble fibers:

Apples	Nuts
Beans	Oat bran
Blueberries	Oats
Carrots	Oranges
Celery	Pears
Cucumbers	Psyllium
Flaxseeds (ground is best)	Strawberries
Lentils	

What About Insoluble Fibers?

As you go about "restoring" healthy gut function, you also have to include foods that are rich in insoluble fibers. These help provide bulk to the stool and prevent constipation. Because these fibers do not dissolve in water, they pass through your gut relatively intact, promoting the passage of food and waste. They are mainly found in whole grains and vegetables.

Sources of Insoluble Fiber

These are among the best sources of insoluble fibers:

Broccoli   Fruits

Brown rice   Green beans

Cabbage   Nuts

Carrots   Seeds

Celery   Whole grains

Cucumbers   Zucchini

Dark, leafy greens

How to take fiber:

Ultimately, for a healthy gut you need a combination of soluble and insoluble fibers. The average American gets only 15 grams (1 tablespoon) of fiber daily in their diet; however, the amount of fiber we should be getting is at least 25 grams (approximately 2 tablespoons) for women and about 35 grams (about ¼ cup) for men. Don't worry about the type of fiber unless you are trying to target a particular health goal, such as lowering your cholesterol, which requires more soluble fiber. Instead, focus on eating foods that span the rainbow of colors. By eating at least nine servings daily of a wide array of different-colored vegetables and fruit in the phytonutrient spectrum—green, yellow, orange, red, blue, deep purple, tan, brown, and white—you will be getting all the soluble and insoluble fibers required for a healthy diet.

HOW TO IMPLEMENT RESTORE DAILY

1. Start with the Gut C.A.R.E. Program RESTORE high-potency once daily probiotic.
2. Look for dairy-free probiotics that contain at least 15 billion CFUs each of *Lactobacillus* and *Bifidobacterium* and take on an empty stomach twice a day for at least three months. For suggestions on quality probiotic supplements, look at the supplement recommendations in Appendix C.
3. Incorporate prebiotic foods into your diet.
4. Add cultured foods, such as the Coconut Water Kefir found in Chapter 9.
5. Incorporate nine total servings of the allowed vegetables and fruit daily.
6. Eat from the phytonutrient spectrum.

ENHANCE

Enhance ⇨ Repair, regenerate, and heal the intestinal lining. *Enhance* digestion, assimilation of nutrients, and gut immune function.

The fourth step of the Gut C.A.R.E. Program is about repairing the damage that has been done to the gut lining—that network of cells forming the interior wall of the intestines that help keep pathogens out, allow nutrients to pass through, and when in a healthy state help keep undigested food particles from being absorbed through the spaces between the cells. For the GI tract to heal and rejuvenate, the right nutritional support is required.

We started the repair process in step one—Cleanse. In that step we removed foods, toxins, and unfavorable microbes that persistently damage the intestinal lining. In step two—Activate—we reintroduced enzymes and nutrients that would assist the mucosa in its healing process. Step three—Restore—focused on providing a healthy microbiota that inhabits every section of our gastrointestinal tract. Now, in the fourth step—Enhance—we will complete this process by restoring the integrity of the tight junctions between the cells of the intestinal lining to keep partially digested food particles, toxins, and microbes from "leaking" into the bloodstream.

THE REPAIR

As prone to injury as the gut lining may be, it also has a tremendous regenerative capacity. In fact, the gut has the largest number of rapidly replicating cells in the body and will repair itself with the right support. When given the opportunity, your body will choose to heal. You just have to provide the favorable environment where this can take place.

You should become familiar with the nutrients that play a pivotal role in the growth, function, repair, and regeneration of the gut mucosa. With these nutrients, you will be able to restore the normal functioning of the cells that line the intestines.

L-Glutamine

L-glutamine is one of the most abundant amino acids in the body and the preferred energy source for the cells that line the small intestine. If glutamine is deficient in the diet, degenerative changes may take place in the small bowel after injuries, such as infections, surgery, stress, and/or radiation. And supplementation with glutamine, an essential component of the Enhance step of the Gut C.A.R.E. Program, has been shown in studies to accelerate the healing of the small intestine, even improving outcomes after whole abdominal radiation.[16] Thus, glutamine is one of the most important nutrients used in the repair process.

How to take L-glutamine:
- Doses start at 1 gram of powder dissolved in water or a capsule on an empty stomach fifteen to twenty minutes before breakfast, lunch, and dinner.

- You can increase the amount as tolerated to 3 grams per dose for a total of 9 grams daily.

- For best delivery to the enterocytes (the cells lining the wall of the intestines), I prefer the powder form. L-glutamine taken between meals can also help curb sugar cravings that arise early on in the program, as you eliminate and detox from all added sugars and any artificial sweeteners in your diet.

DGL (Deglycyrrhizinated Licorice)

Licorice root has been noted to have antiulcer,[17] laxative, anti-inflammatory, immune-modulating, antitumor, and antidiabetic properties.[18,19] And one clinical trial showed its ability to heal eczema when applied topically.[20] Glycyrrhizin is one of the main active ingredients in licorice root, which has favorable liver-protective properties[21] but can also have the negative effect of raising your blood pressure.[22] Deglycyrrhizinated licorice (DGL) is licorice with the glycyrrhizin removed. In terms of the gut, DGL has been shown to protect the stomach lining from damage, even when given to people taking high doses of aspirin, a potent anti-inflammatory that can cause bleeding in the stomach.[23]

How to take DGL:

- DGL can be taken as a chewable tablet before meals for people suffering from gastritis, acid reflux, and indigestion.

- Look for preparations without added sugar.

- 500 milligrams of DGL can also be added in powder form to the L-glutamine powder, along with aloe (discussed below), to make a powerful healing combination for the gut lining.

Aloe Vera

Aloe barbadensis (commonly referred to as aloe vera), a succulent with very thick gelatinous leaves, has been used as a healing plant ever since ancient Egypt, where six-thousand-year-old stone carvings portray the aloe as the "plant of immortality."[24] Aloe offers anti-inflammatory, anti-spasmotic, and cellular protective properties that benefit the gut. In many ways, aloe has been used as a tonic for a variety of ills, including treating constipation, flushing out toxins and waste from the body, and promoting digestion.

ALOE ALLEVIATES STRESS-INDUCED GUT DISTRESS

An animal study of irritable bowel syndrome showed that a combination of aloe vera with German chamomile reduced the severity of stress-induced IBS.[25] And we all know that stress is a big trigger of gut unhappiness. Aloe may also help heal stomach ulcers.[26] The inner gel of the aloe vera plant has even been shown to have antibacterial properties against *H. pylori,* a bacterium that has been implicated as a culprit in stomach ulcers and uncomfortable symptoms of gastritis.[27]

For these reasons, an extract of aloe vera gel powder is an integral part of the Enhance step of the Gut C.A.R.E. Program.

How to take aloe vera:
• Add 100 milligrams to each dose of L-glutamine powder to help enhance its healing action on the digestive lining. The Gut C.A.R.E. Program ENHANCE supplement includes this in a mixture of L-glutamine, DGL, and arabinogalactan from the North American larch tree for the best combination to repair the gut cells. (See Appendix C for more supplement recommendations.)

Essential Fatty Acids

The two main omega-3 fatty acids, EPA (eicosapentaenoic acid) and DHA (docosahexaenoic acid), are important anti-inflammatory promoters in the body that are often deficient in the American diet. Studies have shown that these omega-3s help reduce inflammation in the gut and help reverse mucosal injury.[28,29] Even while increasing omega-3-rich foods in the diet, your body may be in need of an "oil change." The intake of omega-3 fatty acids in the diet over time allows for the exchange of these healthy fats into the cell membrane in place of unhealthy fats that may have been consumed previously, such as trans fats. This facilitates better communication in and out of the cells. This means improved cellular detoxification as waste products are removed and water moves in. This also results in improved signaling, hormone reception, and, in the brain, better communication between neurons.

FISH OIL SUPPLEMENTS

Fish oil supplements usually come in large softgels, and you may need to take a number of capsules to meet the daily requirement. When purchasing an OTC supplement, it's important to read the ingredient list. It may say 1,000 milligrams, but each softgel may contain only 350 milligrams of omega-3 fatty acids per dose. The suggested omega-3 supplements in Appendix C are all high grade, high potency, and devoid of mercury and any other heavy metals and environmental toxins.

How to take omega-3s:

- Take two to four 1,000-milligram softgels daily with meals to enhance their absorption.

- Unless you are vegan or vegetarian, you should also add cold-water fish to your diet to increase your daily intake of omega-3s. For example, a 3-ounce serving of herring or salmon will provide approximately 1.5 grams of omega-3s.

- It is always best to keep omega-3 supplements refrigerated for freshness.

Zinc Carnosine

Zinc deficiency, which is common, can adversely affect the health of the stomach lining and has also been found in individuals with inflammatory diseases of the gut.[30,31] The best test for zinc is a red blood cell zinc, which is only available from certain labs (see Appendix D: Resources).

How to take zinc:
- Take 30 to 50 milligrams daily with food.

- Zinc often needs to be taken with copper at a 20:1 ratio of zinc to copper to maintain proper balance between these trace minerals in the body. (For supplement recommendations see Appendix C.)

HOW TO IMPLEMENT ENHANCE DAILY

1. Start with the Gut C.A.R.E. ENHANCE or an L-glutamine supplement powder mixed with 4 to 8 ounces of water once daily (morning, afternoon, or nighttime) or in your breakfast smoothie.
2. Drink a shot of aloe vera juice every morning. This helps with regularity and reduces gut inflammation.
3. In addition, you may take at least 1 gram of L-glutamine powder three times daily before meals. Increase the amount weekly by 1 gram to a goal of 3 grams before each meal to help reverse your leaky gut.
4. If you suffer from acid reflux or gastritis, take a chewable DGL supplement before meals.
5. Take an omega-3 supplement once or twice daily with meals.
6. If you have symptoms of an upset stomach or stomach ulcer, also take a zinc supplement.

The Gut C.A.R.E. Program is going to be your guide for the next twenty-eight days. It's where you start and a template for you to follow anytime you feel you need to get your health or gut back in order. As a cleanse, it is an excellent program to do at least two or three times a year—for example, to help you lose those holiday pounds in the new year. This is the place where you lay the foundation for healing your gut, reducing the ravages of inflammation in your body, and working your way to a *happy gut* for life. Now get ready for the next twenty-eight days as you prepare to lose your waist and weight at the same time!

A DAY ON THE HAPPY GUT DIET

To make the Gut C.A.R.E. Program as easy to follow as possible, the next few pages are the template for your daily protocol. From sunrise to sundown, I guide you through a day in the Happy Gut Diet. I tell you which supplements to take and how much throughout the day, divided into the times around breakfast, lunch, dinner, and bedtime. I also suggest some gut-friendly snacks to have between meals or as an after-dinner snack, but it's best to stop any snacking one to two hours before you go to bed.

As you can see, supplements are a vital component of the program. They are necessary for you to be successful in C.A.R.E.-ing for your gut. These supplements may be found online at the Happy Gut Life website or at your local health-food store, but I encourage you to research the manufacturers to make sure that you are buying a quality product. Manufacturer quality can vary a great deal, and often what is on the label is not actually in the supplement at the concentrations stated. A list of my recommended companies is provided in the resources section and at www.happygutlife .com. You'll find a supplements checklist at the end of this chapter.

YOUR DAILY PROTOCOL
First Thing in the Morning

- Wake up and set your intention and gratitude for the day. Write down your gratitude in Appendix B.
- Spend five to ten minutes on one yoga pose (see Chapter 8), breathing to connect you with your body.[32]
- Meditate for five minutes: sit in a comfortable position, either cross-legged or on a chair; clear your mind; breathe; center into your body and connect with your core.
- Follow your morning yoga/meditation by squeezing half a lemon into an 8-ounce glass of room temperature or hot water and drink. This routine wakes up your liver and prepares your gut for its digestive functions for the day.

Breakfast

A morning shake with the recommended protein powder and supplements. See the breakfast smoothie recipes in Chapter 9. There are seven recipes for seven days; have each of them, repeat them, or feel free to mix and match as you please. You can even invent your own combinations with the food list in Chapter 2. Try to vary them each day, but always use a hypoallergenic protein powder, such as the Gut C.A.R.E. Cleanse Shake powder, as part of the Gut C.A.R.E. Program.

Supplement Routine

Fifteen to twenty minutes before the morning smoothie with the cup of lemon water:

- 1 complete digestive enzyme support
- 1 high-potency 50 billion CFU multistrain probiotic

With morning smoothie:

- 1 to 2 scoops of hypoallergenic protein powder
- 1 gut-repair powder (1 to 3 grams L-glutamine) dissolved in smoothie
- 2 high-potency omega-3 softgels (approximately 1,500 milligrams)
- 1 plant-based B-complex vitamin/multi-mineral formula[33]
- 1 herbal microbial balancer

Lunch

A meal incorporating the principles of the Happy Gut Diet (Chapters 2, 3, and 4). Chapter 4 will explain how to balance your plate with protein, vegetables, and healthy fats so you can make any meal a gut-healthy meal.

Supplement Routine
Fifteen to twenty minutes before lunch:

- 1 complete digestive enzyme support

With lunch:

- 1 herbal microbial balancer

Snack

Optional, but it will help keep your metabolism moving and keep you from arriving at dinner hungry, which often leads to poor food choices. There is never a reason to feel hungry on the Happy Gut Diet.

Suggested options:

- Raw or steamed vegetables
- Nuts (limit cashews) and seeds (soaked and sprouted are best)[34]

- 1 teaspoon to 1 tablespoon of coconut oil[35] (great source of medium-chain triglycerides to fuel the brain for the end of the workday)
- Green apple wedges* with a nut or seed butter
- Hummus* with raw carrots

*Avoid if you have a FODMAP issue or are on a low-FODMAP diet (explained in Chapter 6).

Dinner

A meal incorporating the principles of the Happy Gut Diet (Chapters 2, 3, and 4), plus supplements. It may be chosen from the recipes in Chapter 9, consisting of a protein with a large salad or vegetable side dish. Take a moment to reflect on your day. Fill in your daily food and symptom diary (Appendix B), and once again express your gratitude for the day. Try to eat dinner at least three hours before going to bed to reduce the chances of acid reflux from undigested food still sitting in your stomach.

Supplement Routine
Fifteen to twenty minutes before dinner:

- 1 complete digestive enzyme support
- 1 gut-repair powder (1 to 3 grams L-glutamine) dissolved in water (this second dose may be taken if you tested positive for leaky gut—see Chapter 6)
- 1 high-potency 50–100 billion CFU multistrain probiotic (this second dose may be taken if you have yeast overgrowth by the self-test on page 176 or extensive gut imbalances as shown in a stool analysis—see Chapter 6)

With dinner:

- 2 high-potency omega-3 softgels (approximately 1,500 milligrams)
- 1 herbal microbial balancer

Post-Dinner Snack

Optional: For those of you who stay up late, you may find that you need an extra something one to two hours before you go to bed. This is when the late-night cravings hit, and the little devil on your shoulder starts suggesting some of the types of foods that got your gut into trouble in the first place. Of course, since you've already done your kitchen cleanse, those are thankfully unavailable. Temptation is strongest when we are stressed or tired, so don't keep temptation nearby.

The fact is, when you crave sweet, your brain isn't necessarily asking for a dessert. Or when you crave salty, your brain isn't necessarily asking for chips. It may be asking for the taste sensation of sweetness, which is best from a natural source. And the salt craving may be asking for something crunchy.

Suggested options:

- Bowl of berries
- 3 celery sticks with nut butter spread on the tips
- 5 green apple wedges* with a thin spread of nut or seed butter

*Avoid if you have a FODMAP issue or are on a low-FODMAP diet (explained in Chapter 6).

After Each Meal

If possible, it is always a good idea to take a five- to ten-minute leisurely walk after each meal to stimulate the digestive process. This is especially important if you work at a desk and spend most of the day sitting. Movement encourages peristalsis (the contractions) of the bowel, clears the mind, and reduces mental tension. Never do strenuous exercise for at least two to three hours after a meal, as it will divert vital blood flow from the intestines to your muscles, leaving the food sitting there undigested and stuck.

Bedtime

A great goal is to end the day with a ten- to fifteen-minute meditation, a little bit longer than the one you started the day with. We'll go into more detail about this in Chapter 8, but for now understand that meditation activates the calming part of the autonomic nervous system, reducing nighttime cravings for sugary or salty snacks and helping you relax before going to sleep. Once you get into this habit, you will find that your sleep is more restful and you will wake up feeling refreshed.

Supplement Routine
Thirty minutes before bed:

- 1 magnesium citrate (200 to 400 milligrams, optional to maintain bowel regularity)*
- 1 triphala[36] (optional)*
- 30 milliliters aloe vera juice or 75 to 300 milligrams gel or resin (optional)*
- Or 1 combination supplement, like the Gut C.A.R.E. RELAX, that contains all three of these supplements

*Optional supplements can be added in a tiered fashion if you suffer from constipation. It is best to work with a health professional to provide guidance on the best combination for you.

SUPPLEMENT CHECKLIST	PURCHASED?
✓ High-potency multistrain probiotic (50+ billion CFUs)	_____
✓ Herbal microbial balancer (berberine, 250 to 500 milligrams)	_____
✓ Combo gut-repair powder (L-glutamine, DGL, aloe)	_____
✓ *Or* L-glutamine powder alone (1 to 3 grams)	_____
✓ Hypoallergenic protein powder	_____
✓ Complete digestive enzyme support	_____
✓ High-potency omega-3 fish oil	_____
✓ Magnesium citrate +/- triphala +/- aloe	_____
✓ Plant-based B complex vitamin/multi-mineral formula[37]	_____

See Appendix C and visit www.happygutlife.com for more suggestions on how to live with a happy gut.

4

TIPS FOR SUCCESS: CREATING A HAPPY GUT

Now THAT YOU UNDERSTAND the Gut C.A.R.E. Program, it's time to put it into action. During the next twenty-eight days you will eliminate from your diet the most common foods that result in food sensitivities or immune reactions, water retention, and weight gain. Remember, these issues are caused by the foods you eat on a daily basis that lead to an immune response in your gut without your realizing it. This also interferes with your metabolism. It may seem unfair that the top foods that short-circuit your gut happiness and weight-loss attempts also happen to be some of the most predominant foods in human diets worldwide. But trust that you can do this.

The first three to seven days, as you cut out the most troublesome high-sensitivity foods from your diet, will be the hardest. In this chapter you will learn what it's like to get started on the Happy Gut Diet, along with typical troubleshooting questions.

First, let's look at two weeks on the Happy Gut Diet by considering a sample meal plan.

THE HAPPY GUT MEAL PLAN

When putting together any meal plan, the most important thing is to select foods you really enjoy. Throughout the twenty-eight-day Gut C.A.R.E. Program, you can choose from many of the recipes I created with the Happy Gut chefs as well as additional selections listed below. I want you to feel nourished, not deprived, so this plan has been designed so that you never need to feel hungry or "on a diet," with enough healthy, gut-friendly snacks you can reach for when you need one between meals. Being happy with your choices makes it easy and fun to stay on track to heal your gut and lose weight.

You should select three meals and two or three optional snacks spaced evenly throughout the day. The recipes are arranged with Monday as Day 1, but you can choose to begin any day of the week that works for you. It is okay to repeat a particular selection if you like it. Feel free to add additional steamed vegetables or seasonings from the allowed food lists to any of the suggestions below. Recipes marked with an asterisk (*) can be found in the *Happy Gut* recipe collection in Chapter 9.

I reserved recipes that require more preparation for the weekends, based on a Monday start. To save time during your busy workweek, you can prepare a few recipes over the weekend. Soups can easily be frozen for later use. You can also cut vegetables on the weekend and have them ready to go when you need them for a salad or a healthy go-to snack.

YOUR DAILY PLAN

EVERY DAY

A.M. Starter
8 ounces of room temperature or hot water with half a squeezed lemon

	Breakfast	Snack	Lunch	Afternoon Snack	Dinner	Snack
DAY 1	Matcha Energizer Smoothie*	Organic green apple slices with a nut or seed butter spread	Buckwheat Pasta and Vegetables in Homemade Vegetable Broth*	Veggie sticks with hummus	Chicken Piccata* served with roasted or steamed vegetables	Mint tea
DAY 2	Swiss Chard and Strawberry Smoothie*	Plain coconut yogurt with organic blueberries	Free-range baked turkey cutlets served with sliced avocado over steamed spinach	Hummus with Flax Super-Seed Crackers*	Roasted Free-Range Chicken* over mixed greens (save leftovers)	Herbal tea
DAY 3	Raspberry Recharge Smoothie*	Crispy Kale Chips*	Chicken Curry* with brown rice and steamed vegetables	Flax Super-Seed Crackers* with sunflower seed butter	Baked acorn squash, sliced and topped with dairy-free coconut yogurt and sprinkled with toasted pumpkin seeds	Coconut Water Kefir*
DAY 4	Spicy Avocado Smoothie*	Veggie sticks	Roasted Free-Range Chicken* slices (from Day 2) on organic mesclun greens with Dr. Pedre's Scallion Vinaigrette*	Nut and Seed Bar*	Beef Kabobs* served with additional steamed vegetables	Small bowl of organic berries

	Breakfast	Snack	Lunch	Afternoon Snack	Dinner	Snack
DAY 5	Go Green Smoothie*	Green tea with lemon	Wild low-mercury tuna marinated in olive oil, lemon, cilantro, salt, and pepper on a bed of organic baby greens	Flax Super-Seed Crackers* with homemade guacamole	Stuffed Mexican Turkey Burger* with Cilantro Pesto* and greens	Organic green apple slices or herbal tea
DAY 6	Blue Ginger Smoothie*	Grass-Fed Beef-Bone Broth*	Roasted Wild Salmon with Dill Sauce* served with organic baby greens and Dr. Pedre's Scallion Vinaigrette*	Veggie sticks with hummus	Chicken Curry* served with organic basmati brown rice	2 Almond-Hemp Chocolate Truffles*
DAY 7	Chocolate-Covered Almond Protein Smoothie *	Organic baby carrots	Chicken and Pistachio Lettuce Wraps*	Mediterranean Chickpea Salad*	Mahi-Mahi with Shallots, Lime, and Veggies in Parchment*	1 Coconut Macaroon*
DAY 8	Go Green Smoothie*	Green tea with lemon	Chopped salad of organic mixed greens, cucumbers, avocado, carrots, beets, and Roasted Free-Range Chicken* with olive oil, apple cider vinegar, salt, and pepper	Quinoa Salad with Apples and Walnuts*	Stir-Fried Veggies and Shrimp over Rice Noodles*	Small bowl of organic mixed berries or herbal tea

	Breakfast	Snack	Lunch	Afternoon Snack	Dinner	Snack
DAY 9	Swiss Chard and Strawberry Smoothie*	Organic green apple	Summer Fresh Citrus Salad with Sliced Almonds* (optional: add organic grilled chicken or Roasted Free-Range Chicken* slices from Day 2)	Nut and Seed Bar*	Roasted Wild Salmon with Dill Sauce* served with organic baby greens and Dr. Pedre's Scallion Vinaigrette*	Mint tea
DAY 10	Blue Ginger Smoothie*	Coconut Water Kefir*	Grilled strips of organic zucchini (marinated in olive oil, sea salt, lemon juice, and garlic) served with chickpeas	Fresh berries with chopped walnuts	Bison Burger* served with Roasted Sweet Potato Wedges with Toasted Pumpkin Seeds*	Grass-Fed Beef-Bone Broth* (cold or warm)
DAY 11	Matcha Energizer Smoothie*	Crispy Kale Chips*	Summer Fresh Citrus Salad with Sliced Almonds* with Veggie-Stuffed Spring Rolls*	Veggie sticks with hummus	Seared Steak with Dijon-Horseradish Sauce* served with roasted organic sweet potatoes or a side salad	Small organic green apple baked with a sprinkle of cinnamon and chopped walnuts
DAY 12	Spicy Avocado Smoothie*	Nut and Seed Bar*	Harvest Wild Rice Bowl*	Green tea with lemon	Roasted Free-Range Chicken* over organic mesclun greens	Fresh Berries with Whipped Coconut Cream*

	Breakfast	Snack	Lunch	Afternoon Snack	Dinner	Snack
DAY 13	Raspberry Recharge Smoothie*	Vanilla rooibos tea	Mixed green salad with poached wild salmon, sliced cucumbers, black olives, and dill	Butternut Squash Bisque with Toasted Walnuts*	Rosemary Lamb* and Roasted Cauliflower with Toasted Walnuts Topping*	Herbal tea
DAY 14	Chocolate-Covered Almond Protein Smoothie*	Veggie sticks	Mediterranean Chickpea Salad* with Flax Super-Seed Crackers*	Grass-Fed Beef-Bone Broth*	Chicken and Pistachio Lettuce Wraps*	Organic green apple slices with almond butter or herbal tea

DETOXING FROM YOUR FOOD SENSITIVITIES AND ADDICTIONS

During the first week of the program, you may experience detox reactions from not eating foods that were telling your brain it wanted more of them, even while they were causing pain and inflammation and zapping you of energy. It seems counterintuitive that getting rid of these foods will actually make you feel worse at first, but that is often the case. Your body will experience withdrawal symptoms, similar to detoxing from an addictive substance. For a few days, your cravings for those foods may also increase. Your willpower will be challenged. You may suffer from headaches, mental fog, fatigue, achiness, joint pains, and general malaise. Your symptoms may even seem to get worse. This is your body processing out the inflammatory foods that have been activating your immune system. These foods were making you sick without your realizing it!

FOOD ANTIGEN –
IMMUNE COMPLEXES

Food antigens are food protein particles that stimulate the immune
system when you have a leaky gut. This diagram shows how your body
clears food antigens by following the food elimination in the Happy
Gut Diet. You start to feel less sick as the immune system quiets down.

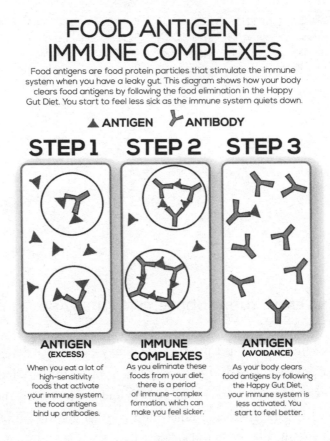

▲ ANTIGEN   Ⓨ ANTIBODY

STEP 1   STEP 2   STEP 3

ANTIGEN
(EXCESS)

When you eat a lot of
high-sensitivity
foods that activate
your immune system,
the food antigens
bind up antibodies.

IMMUNE
COMPLEXES

As you eliminate these
foods from your diet,
there is a period
of immune-complex
formation, which can
make you feel sicker.

ANTIGEN
(AVOIDANCE)

As your body clears
food antigens by following
the Happy Gut Diet,
your immune system is
less activated. You
start to feel better.

As your immune system breaks down the protein molecules that have
turned it on, it goes through a period of high alert. Once these protein
antigens have been processed and released, your immune cells will begin
to quiet down; internal inflammation will decrease; you will feel less
achy, less swollen, and less bloated; and your head will become clearer.

The Gut C.A.R.E. Program is designed to support your body
through this process by reinforcing detox pathways so you can get
through it as easily as possible. In other words, with a Gut C.A.R.E.
morning breakfast smoothie, your liver, kidneys, and (most important)

intestines will be able to handle the detox load that they will experience at the beginning of the program. You will not only be shedding toxins from your body, but you will also be getting rid of the excess water you retained because of inflammation, losing the bloated feeling. As a result, you will naturally lose weight without counting calories. It's that simple.

HOW TO EAT

How we eat is just as important as what we eat. Our eating philosophy not only factors into our food choices but also into how our body digests and assimilates foods. Some general principles for eating will help you eat only the right amount, keep you feeling satisfied with each meal, and improve the entire digestive process.

Social Eating

When your gut is unhappy and unpredictable, you often choose to remove the social aspect of eating from your life. It's uncomfortable and embarrassing to have to excuse yourself in the middle of a restaurant meal with friends or while on a date because your bowels are acting up. During the next twenty-eight days of the Happy Gut Diet, it's time to reconnect to the roots of eating. Throughout history, eating has been a shared experience, enriched as much by the company as it is by the food.

Conscious Eating

When you eat, slow down. Take in the conversation. How often have you been eating something as if in a daze when you suddenly realize that you just ate through the entire plate in five minutes? Eating in conscious, positive engagement with others permits you to savor the flavors, and it promotes the internal relaxation that stimulates the digestive process so it can run smoothly. After all, digestion is designed to occur in a relaxed state, and it is hindered by agitation, stress, rushing, and eating on the go.

Even if you are eating alone, taking a moment to express gratitude for the food you are about to consume and nourish your body with changes the dynamic immediately. It brings eating into the realm of consciousness. You will naturally slow down, chew thoroughly, savor the flavors, and promote the parasympathetic nervous response that accepts the food in your gut without distress.

Filling Your Plate: The One-Quarter/Three-Quarters Rule

When filling your plate with food, imagine that it is divided into quarters. Fill one-quarter of your plate with protein and healthy, omega-3-rich fats (wild-caught fatty fish, grass-fed meats, humanely raised and antibiotic-free chicken, avocado, etc.), and fill the other three-quarters with greens and veggies (raw, baked, or steamed). This simple rule will ensure that you get the right balance of proteins, fats, and carbs without the stress of having to weigh your food or count calories. Now you can simply enjoy the act of eating.

Here's another rule of thumb: never let your food touch the edges of the plate. In other words, don't fill your plate so full that it is overflowing. If you are trying to eat smaller portions, serve yourself with a smaller plate, still adhering to the 1:3 proportion of protein to vegetables. This will help reduce the amount of food you eat at one time, giving your stomach and brain the opportunity to realize you are full. We will talk more about satiety shortly.

Chewing Your Food

As we discussed in Chapter 2, digestion begins in the mouth. As you chew your food, your saliva mixed with the mechanically broken-down food particles begins the digestive process. You should chew food so that it becomes a soft pulp in your mouth before you swallow. This may take a different number of chews depending on the consistency of what you are eating. Some foods are softer and will require less chewing, and others will require more chewing to make them digestible.

When you swallow, this mass of food and saliva moves through your esophagus into the acidic environment of the stomach for further breakdown. The stomach is where the very important process of breaking down proteins into amino acids takes place. Your body utilizes these amino acids for the repair and building of tissues as well as the production of enzymes and neurotransmitters. Before the food gets to your stomach, remember that the better you masticate (chew food into pieces), the easier it will be for the stomach to do its job.

MINIMIZE DRINKING WHILE YOU EAT

If you chew your food thoroughly, you will produce enough saliva mixed with the food that you will not need to drink any fluids during a meal. This may sound counterintuitive, especially when any time you eat out, you are offered a beverage.

If you do have a drink, avoid drinking excessively while eating so that you don't dilute your stomach acid. Instead, drink water between meals, or wait until fifteen to thirty minutes after the meal to drink fluids, as this will make digesting food easier for your body. Yes, it is important to get at least 64 ounces (approximately eight glasses) of water daily, but drink most of it before or between meals.

Remember, if you need to have a drink to help you swallow your food, you're probably eating too fast, swallowing air with your food, and not chewing enough. This will cause stomach bloating and discomfort in your upper abdomen.

Swallowing and Satiety

Swallow your food patiently. Don't gulp it down. When you gulp your food, you swallow air with your food, which then distends your stomach and makes you feel uncomfortable. If you suffer from acid reflux, it's important to remember this and to eat smaller, more frequent meals. Slowing down to chew sufficiently and swallow patiently are key ways to avoid overeating.

When to Stop

Learn to recognize when you are almost 75 percent full and stop eating after a few more bites. Wait a few minutes to see if you are really still hungry. More often than not, you will have reached your capacity. If you keep eating after that point, you are eating with your mind, possibly your eyes, but not your visceral senses. Learn how to listen to those "gut feelings" in more ways than one, and you will master the art of eating just the right amount for yourself.

AN EXERCISE IN MINDFUL EATING

Place a blueberry in your mouth. Don't bite it; just let it sit there on your tongue or between your teeth. Observe it. What does it feel like? What are the textures? Is there a flavor? Take a moment to experience this, then bite into it. What happens next? The softness inside of the blueberry releases. More intense flavors light up your taste buds. The interior pulp is moist on your tongue. There are sweet tones mixed with the tartness of the outer skin. There is so much more happening that we are usually oblivious to when we eat. You can do this experiment with all types of foods. Try this at the family dinner table. Ask others to share their experiences. Bring your senses to your food.

YOUR LIFESTYLE AND A HAPPY GUT

Most of us don't give much consideration to the way we live our daily lives because it has become normal for us. However, normal may mean being in a rush all the time, eating quick meals at a work desk, habitually ruminating over work or life stresses, and not taking the time to engage in self-care that is so necessary for a balanced life and a healthy, happy gut.

Getting Proper Sleep

Insomnia in any form, whether it's difficulty falling asleep, staying asleep, or both, disturbs your body's delicate internal rhythms. Anyone who has had a run of sleepless nights also knows that it leads to increased anxiety. Eventually, you may feel wired while feeling exhausted at the same time. This will throw off your gut rhythm, leading to either constipation or diarrhea.

Working the night shift is another major problem. The later you stay up, the more you crave something sweet or starchy. Your body is tired, and it wants quick energy to keep it going. By the next morning, the digestive system is out of sync, and eating can actually make you feel sick to your stomach. If you are a shift worker, some of this is out of your control. For most of us, though, the choice to have regular sleep times is ours to make.

I cannot stress enough the importance of regular sleep patterns. Consistency is key, as the body and your gut like predictability.

Reducing Stress

Stress is a major and underestimated factor that affects the gut, even when all other lifestyle behaviors (diet and exercise) are on point. Stress increases inflammation, regardless of how good you're being with your diet. It activates the fight-or-flight response that makes you feel like you're under attack when you're not. It can lead to elevated blood pressure, palpitations, and reduced blood flow to the intestines, resulting in poor digestion and assimilation of nutrients.

Some live under and handle such elevated levels of stress on a daily basis that they consider it normal. They've ceased to notice what a huge impact stress has on their lives and their gut function, as if they have become desensitized to stress. I often point out to my patients how full their plates are and how even if the load they carry (between work and social life) feels "normal," it shouldn't be their "normal."

Stress can exacerbate any and all of the symptoms we experience in our bodies. In Chapter 8, I'll offer ways you can use yoga and breath work to reduce your stress response and create a more wholesome life for yourself with a happier gut.

HAPPY GUT FAQs

These are some of the more common questions I'm asked by patients:

Q: I'm feeling great after twenty-one days on the Happy Gut Diet; can I transition sooner into the Reintroduction Phase?

A: The short answer is, you shouldn't. If you transition early, even if you are feeling well, you have not allowed enough time for your food sensitivities to calm down, and you may trigger a more vigorous immune reaction to the foods you reintroduce. Allow your gut time to cool off and heal on the Gut C.A.R.E. regimen. When it comes to the gut, shortcuts do not pay off.

Q: I've completed the twenty-eight-day Happy Gut Diet. Now what?

A: After the twenty-eight days, you may begin the Reintroduction Phase (discussed in Chapter 5). This is where you challenge yourself with the foods we eliminated during the Happy Gut Diet. If the food challenge causes new symptoms or some of your old ones to come back, then you should stay on the Happy Gut Diet and the Gut C.A.R.E. Program for at least three months, possibly six months. This ensures that the greatest amount of healing will occur.

Q: *I feel like I'm running out of things to eat. What do I do?*

A: Whenever you start any new eating plan, you may tend to streamline your diet into a few items that are familiar. This can make for an easy transition when planning your meals initially, but eventually you get bored with your options. There is no reason for this to happen, because the options in the Happy Gut Diet are varied. Revisit the meal plan on pages 118–121 for guidance as to how to vary your meals. Try something you have never tried before. Try one of the recipes in Chapter 9—choose one that makes you feel slightly uncomfortable because it has ingredients you don't normally eat or cook with. This is an opportunity to expand your eating palate.

Q: *I'm experiencing frequent acid reflux. How can I reduce it naturally?*

A: Here are helpful tips for reducing and eliminating symptoms of acid reflux or indigestion:

TEN HELPFUL TIPS TO REDUCE ACID REFLUX

1. Avoid carbonated beverages before or during your meals.
2. Chew your food well. Eat slowly to avoid swallowing excessive air with your food that will then increase the pressure inside your stomach.
3. Avoid eating the most common foods that lead to acid reflux. These include:
   • Coffee/caffeine (although herbal, black, and green teas may be okay)
   • Acidic juices (like orange juice)
   • Alcohol (especially acidic wines)

- Fried foods
- Tomato sauces/ketchup
- Dairy/cheeses
- Spicy foods (hot spices, like curry and cayenne)
- Sautéed onions
- Chocolate
- Mint

4. Eat at least three hours before bedtime; don't eat dinner and then lie down to sleep.
5. Quit smoking. Smoking relaxes the lower esophageal sphincter, which leads to more reflux.
6. Don't chew gum excessively.
7. Keep a food and symptom diary to uncover acid reflux triggers. Food triggers may be unique to you.
8. Drink plenty of water between meals, but not during meals. I recommend at least 64 ounces daily, adjusted to your activity and weather conditions.
9. Take a digestive enzyme (see Appendix C for suggestions) fifteen minutes before meals as an alternative therapy for your reflux symptoms. You can do this from one to four weeks, depending on the severity of your symptoms, or even keep one on hand when you know you're going to eat a particularly challenging meal.
10. Avoid taking OTC medications for more than two weeks without speaking to your doctor or health-care practitioner.

Q: *What happens to my gut when I travel? Is it normal for it to behave differently?*

A: Although people don't expect their gut to behave differently when traveling, it usually will. When traveling, the digestive system is thrown out of rhythm more often than not. The most common disturbance when people travel is constipation.

The reasons your gut gets out of sync when traveling are:

1. **Increased physical activity:** You are a lot more active while traveling (walking more), meaning you sweat more, which dehydrates your body and makes the stool harder. Harder stools have a tougher time getting through the colon.
2. **Dehydration:** You tend to drink less water, and water is necessary to keep the stool at the right consistency to travel through the intestines. Flying is very dehydrating. Alcoholic beverages are also dehydrating, and drinking them while on vacation makes for fun but worsens your constipation.
3. **Less fiber:** You tend to eat less fiber and more foods that will slow down your gut transit.
4. **More bread:** You go off your healthy diet and eat more bread, which forms a thick mass in your intestines. This stubborn mass does not want to move.
5. **Disturbed sleep:** Your circadian rhythm is disturbed when you travel, especially between time zones. This throws off the delicate internal rhythm of your enteric (gut) nervous system (discussed in Chapter 7), which leads to more constipation. Try to eat lighter meals at the time you would normally eat your meals, but in the new time zone, to coax your gut back into rhythm.

Q: What are the best strategies and remedies to alleviate constipation?

A: A backed-up gut is an unhappy gut, which makes for an unhappy person. The retained stool is full of toxins that have to exit your body, so the goal is to have at least one bowel movement daily. Some people may have up to three bowel movements daily, one after each meal, but most suffer from constant or intermittent constipation.

Here are the best strategies for dealing with constipation:

1. **Hydration:** The first and most important treatment for constipation is to make sure that you are drinking at least 64 fluid ounces of water daily and don't dehydrate with caffeine.

2. **Fiber:** Make sure you are eating the daily recommended amount of fiber (see page 102).

3. **Magnesium citrate:** This type of magnesium salt safely helps draw more water into the stool to keep it moving. Start with 200 milligrams at bedtime and increase the dose by 100 to 200 milligrams every other day until you find the dosage that works for you. You may find that it works best to take it in the morning.

4. **Buffered vitamin C powder:** When taken at a high enough dose, vitamin C will promote a bowel movement, but this treatment is best reserved for when you have been severely constipated and nothing is working. Start with 1,000 milligrams of buffered vitamin C, and keep taking 1,000 milligrams once every hour until you have a bowel movement. Keep a record of the dose you reach and make that your special constipation rescue dose.

5. **Triphala:** An Indian ayurvedic blend that balances all body types, allowing for easy digestion and bowel movements. For best results, you should take this on a daily basis.

6. **Psyllium husks:** A type of fiber that comes from the outer coating of psyllium seeds. It is a soluble fiber that helps promote bowel movements when taken with plenty of water. However, you do not want to take too much of this fiber. A study done on patients with a history of colorectal adenomas (a type of benign tumor with the potential to become malignant) found that the soluble fiber from the psyllium husk increased the risk of recurrence of colorectal adenomas by 67 percent.[1]

7. **Senna:** A natural laxative derived from the leaves of the senna plant. It irritates the lining of the intestines to promote bowel movements, but when used excessively it can lead to dependence. Depending on a laxative to have a bowel movement disturbs your gut's delicate internal rhythm. Only use senna occasionally for constipation when you are really backed up, but not on a regular basis.

Except for the last two (psyllium and senna), the other remedies are safe to use on a regular basis to maintain bowel regularity. Vary the dose of your remedy depending on how you are feeling and how your diet has been.

Q: *Are there herbal teas to soothe an upset stomach?*

A: Herbal teas that soothe an upset stomach and reduce nausea include chamomile, ginger, and fennel. Two of my favorites are Stomach Ease and Ginger by Yogi Tea. I sip these plain or add 1 teaspoon of honey to soften the bitterness. To make a stronger, more medicinal tea, simply steep the tea bag for up to ten minutes. For a more powerful nerve- and gut-soothing chamomile, purchase dried chamomile flower pods at a health-food store, bring to a boil in a pot, then simmer for ten to fifteen minutes. You can drink it warm or make a refreshing iced chamomile tea with a sprig of fresh mint leaf.

For more answers to your questions, visit www.happygutlife.com.

The next section will continue to explore ways you can incorporate the concepts in *Happy Gut* for the rest of your life. We will look at how you transition out of the twenty-eight-day Happy Gut Diet into the Reintroduction Phase. In Chapter 6, I will give you guidance on how to address any gut issues that may arise immediately or in the future.

PART III

REINTRODUCTION PHASE
AND FURTHER TESTING

REINTRODUCTION AND YOUR GUT C.A.R.E. PLAN FOR LIFE

W ITH EXPOSURES TO DIFFERENT foods, travel, medications, antibiotics, environmental toxins, and dietary indiscretions (like too much sugar over the holidays), you'll certainly experience ups and downs with your gut function. When you get off track you can always return to the basics in Chapter 3 to C.A.R.E.—Cleanse, Activate, Restore, and Enhance—for your gut. We all slip up from time to time, and that's okay. You'll have the tools in *Happy Gut* to help you rebalance your gut and regain your health each time you need to.

THE REINTRODUCTION PHASE

In the Reintroduction Phase of the diet, you get to add back foods you were not eating in Phase I. During Reintroduction, you will need to be a keen observer of how your body reacts when you again eat the high-sensitivity foods you have been avoiding.

Reintroduce foods *in the following order*:

1. Organic, free-range eggs: Start with boiled, poached, or steamed sunny-side-up eggs, or egg white omelets. Avoid scrambled eggs or

whole-egg omelets at first; they are harder to digest because of the oil added during preparation.

2. Organic, rBGH-free dairy: Start with cultured dairy products (like plain yogurt and kefirs). You may also add raw-milk cheese or goat cheese. Avoid sweetened (artificial or not) yogurts and flavored yogurts and kefirs, which will inevitably contain added sugar. Making your own at home is the best.

3. Non-GMO corn[1]

4. Non-GMO fermented soy (like tempeh or miso)

5. Legumes[2]

6. Wheat/gluten

You will reintroduce one food every four days, starting with the first. Eat the food more than once on the introduction day to challenge your gut and your body. If no symptoms are apparent, rechallenge with the food the next day for breakfast.

If you experience a recurrence of old symptoms or the onset of new symptoms within the first twenty-four to thirty-six hours (for example, you feel fatigued, mentally foggy, sleepy, achy, stiff, etc.), that food group should be placed back on the "avoid" list. If, after two days, you do not experience any new symptoms when you reintroduce a food item, give yourself another two days to simply observe for any reactions that may have been delayed. After four days you will reintroduce the next food. If you don't react to a reintroduced food, you may add it back into your diet, but don't add new foods more than two times per week to avoid overexposure to a high-sensitivity food.

This is how it looks:

DAY 1	Introduce eggs	Record any new symptoms or recurrence of old symptoms
DAY 2	Rechallenge eggs*	Record any new symptoms or recurrence of old symptoms
DAY 3	Avoid	Observe how you feel
DAY 4	Avoid	Observe how you feel
DAY 5	Introduce dairy	Record any new symptoms or recurrence of old symptoms
DAY 6	Rechallenge dairy**	Record any new symptoms or recurrence of old symptoms
DAY 7	Avoid	Observe how you feel
DAY 8	Avoid all or eat eggs if no reaction	Observe how you feel

*Only rechallenge if you do not experience new or old symptoms on day 1.
**Only rechallenge if you do not experience new or old symptoms on day 5.

. . . and so on.

Not everyone will have had an issue with nightshades. If nightshades were eliminated during your first twenty-eight days, you will need twenty-eight days, rather than twenty-four, to complete the entire Reintroduction Phase.

WHAT ABOUT SUGAR DURING THIS PHASE?

Notice I didn't mention reintroducing sugar. Sugar is at the root of much of the energy-sapping, inflammatory, mood-disturbing toxicity of foods. Artificial sweeteners should never be reintroduced. Agave, a natural alternative sweetener often touted as healthier because of its low-glycemic effects, is a dangerous alternative sweetener that is no better than high-fructose corn syrup. Adding back limited amounts of honey, maple syrup, and cane sugar as sweeteners is acceptable, but only incrementally. Desserts should be an occasional treat (no more than twice per week) in concordance with the part of the reintroduction phase you are in. If you have a history of *Candida* or recurrent yeast infections, sugar will have to be markedly limited for up to six months or possibly longer. With fruits that were not allowed in the Happy Gut Diet, it's best to choose seasonal offerings and no more than two servings daily.

If you continue to react to the high-sensitivity foods discussed in previous chapters (with symptoms that include weight gain, pain, or bloating), my best advice is to continue to avoid those foods for three months (from the day you started the Happy Gut Diet). Although this will be challenging, in the long run you will be grateful that you did so. In the meantime, you may continue to rotate the nonreactive foods in your diet every three to four days. This means that you do not eat the same foods day after day.

At the beginning of the fourth month, rechallenge your gut with those high-sensitivity foods using the methods described above, carefully observing how you feel after eating the food. If you again have apparent symptoms, then avoid that food for another three months before rechallenging. Allowing a longer cool-off period for your immune system while healing your leaky gut is the best way to minimize the effects these foods were having on you.

If Your Gut Becomes Unhappy Again

If you still react negatively to all the foods, you should stay on the Happy Gut Diet and the Gut C.A.R.E. Program supplements to heal your gut, and go on to Chapter 6 to learn what tests will be helpful in uncovering your root causes. Don't despair—with time, as you heal your leaky gut, you will be able to reintroduce foods and not have a reaction. However, you may need to continue to avoid one or more categories because they persistently aggravate your digestive system or worsen your gut-associated conditions. As hard as this may seem at the beginning, when my patients realize how great they feel by continuing to avoid these foods, the choice in favor of their health over indulgence is easy to make.

YOUR GUT C.A.R.E. PLAN FOR LIFE

By now, you should have a clear understanding of which foods are agreeable to your gut and which foods still cause digestive or body-wide symptoms. While I have given you the tools to complete this process on your own, it is always helpful to work with your health-care practitioner, a nutritionist, or a health coach to help you understand and interpret any symptoms that may arise. At www.happygutlife.com, we can connect you to a health coach to work with you as you embark on this life-changing journey.

One important thing to bear in mind about the gut is that it changes over time depending on what you are putting into your body. The cleansing program provided here is meant to make you aware of how much more control you have over this than you previously realized. As you look toward how you will continue to eat after you have completed the Gut C.A.R.E. Program, keep in mind all the principles of the Happy Gut Diet.

CLEANSING TO STAY HEALTHY

Cleansing is a great way to keep your digestive system and your body vibrant, energetic, and healthy. It promotes cellular rejuvenation by removing toxins and adding the right types of nutrients. You may also find there are periods during which you feel better by taking out all or a few of the high-sensitivity foods from your diet. Repeating the Happy Gut cleansing program twice a year is a great way to do this. It is like hitting the "reboot" button for your gut and body after a period of not eating as healthfully.

You have to continuously adapt to the changing conditions in your gut—tuning in to hunger signals as well as maintaining a balance between heavier meals and lighter meals. Do not eat just because it's time to eat. Consume food because you are hungry, and eat only the amount that nourishes you. The principles discussed in Chapter 4 should continue to guide the way you eat in the future.

FURTHER TESTING FOR GUT-RELATED AILMENTS

L IKE JULIE, WHOM WE met in the Introduction, you may have been at your breaking point. You've been suffering from GI distress or related body symptoms for a long time and have lost faith that there is any hope for relief. You may have been placed on a medication that masks the symptoms without addressing the underlying root causes.

If not for the combination of standard Western tests and the functional tests I am going to discuss in this chapter, Julie would have continued suffering with a diagnosis of "IBS," and she could have been written off as one of those patients who simply never recover. Instead, the standard and functional tests I ran on Julie allowed us to uncover the root causes, treat them, and support her body in its ability to heal and recover from chronic illness.

HOW TO USE THIS CHAPTER

This chapter is full of diagnostic tests and conditions you may or may not have heard of before. It is a lot of information, so you may want to skim through it initially to get an idea of what the different gut imbalances are and how they are diagnosed. You do not need to know your own unique imbalances to begin the Happy Gut Diet and Gut C.A.R.E. Program;

however, these tests can help you further refine and guide you toward gut and total body wellness. Don't be overwhelmed by the amount of information here, as this chapter is meant to be a reference you can use to help you work with your health practitioner to uncover what condition(s) underlie your symptoms or any new symptoms that arise. If your symptoms return after the Reintroduction Phase, the tests in this chapter are the next step in achieving total body wellness.

I have taken great care to simplify the testing menu to make it accessible to you with bulleted symptom lists, charts, and descriptions on how to test for each condition, but there are still many details I may not have included here. Even more specific details about each condition and testing are available at www.happygutlife.com.

TEN COMMON AND NOT-SO-COMMON
TESTS EVERYONE SHOULD HAVE

No matter what your underlying issues, there are routine tests that are meant to pick up on general abnormalities related to gut health. These are the tests (with their medical terminology) so you know what to ask to be tested for:

1. **CBC (Complete Blood Count).** This tests for white and red blood cell characteristics and platelet count. An iron deficiency will show up as anemia— a low hemoglobin and/or lower production of red blood cells.

2. **Iron Profile with Ferritin.** This test is the best way to measure for an iron deficiency. Low ferritin means that body stores of iron are low. This may be due to blood loss from menstruation but can signify something more serious, like internal bleeding in the gut. Low iron may also mean that there is inadequate absorption because of low stomach acidity. High ferritin is a sign of inflammation, often seen in autoimmune conditions like rheumatoid arthritis and lupus, and may exist in combination with an anemia because chronic inflammation disrupts red blood cell production.

3. **Fasting Glucose.** This is a measure of how much sugar (glucose) is present in your blood after an overnight fast. The goal is for a level <90 mg/dl, even

though normal is considered less than 100 mg/dl. Between 100 and 125 mg/dl is considered insulin resistance or prediabetes. If your level is ≥126 mg/dl, then you are diabetic, but a random nonfasting glucose >140 mg/dl is also diagnostic. Diabetes can lead to gastroparesis—a condition marked by postprandial fullness because the stomach does not empty as quickly as it should.

4. **CMP (Complete Metabolic Profile).** This is a routine measure of electrolytes and liver, gallbladder, and kidney function. In reference to the gut, we are specifically looking for disturbances in liver and gallbladder function that could signify a reduced ability to detoxify through your liver or gallbladder. Liver inflammation can show up as elevated liver enzymes (known as transaminases—ALT and AST for short). Elevated liver enzymes may result from fat buildup in your liver (a.k.a. fatty liver) when your diet is too high in sugar (including high-fructose corn syrup) and refined carbohydrates.

5. **Amylase/Lipase.** This is a useful screening tool for inflammation of the pancreas (the endocrine gland where lipase, the fat-digestion enzyme, and insulin, the sugar-regulating hormone, are produced). An elevated amylase or lipase means that something is injuring the pancreas. However, neither of these markers reveals anything about pancreatic function. See functional markers of pancreatic function later in the chapter.

6. **Insulin Level.** Insulin is a peptide hormone produced in the beta cells of the pancreas and helps us use sugar (glucose) for energy. When you eat a meal that has sugar or carbohydrates, the glucose in the meal triggers the release of insulin. However, when you eat too much sugar or simple starches, excessive amounts of insulin are secreted, eventually leading to insulin resistance and the storage of fat around your belly. The best way to measure insulin is to check a fasting insulin level. Aim for <5 mg/dl or a fasting glucose-to-insulin ratio >7.0, as long as the fasting glucose is in an optimal range (see number 3).

7. **Thyroid Function Tests (TFTs).** The most commonly ordered thyroid function test is the TSH (thyroid stimulating hormone).[1] Symptoms of a sluggish thyroid include hair loss, thinning hair, brittle nails, constipation, fatigue, mental slowness, and dry skin. However, many people with subclinical hypothyroidism may have a normal TSH with subnormal thyroid hormones. The hormones produced by the thyroid include T4 and T3. Each of these travels in both a form bound to blood proteins (like albumin and thyroglobulin) that carry it through your circulatory system (the total value) and the free form. T4 is like the savings account, and T3 is

like the actual currency that exerts its effects on the body. For your body to make T3, T4 needs to be converted to T3 by the enzyme 5'-deiodinase, which relies on the trace mineral selenium as a cofactor. If selenium is deficient in your diet, you can have hypothyroid symptoms with a normal TSH simply because conversion of T4 to T3 is affected.

8. **Thyroid Antibodies.** Because of their connection to dietary soy and gluten, thyroid antibody tests are an important screening tool when customizing nutritional changes that can have a significant impact on your long-term health. See Chapter 2 for more information.

9. **Vitamin D.** Not a vitamin but actually a hormone, vitamin D is of utmost importance in regulating the immune response in addition to increasing calcium absorption in the gut and mobilizing it to the bones. The active form, 1,25-OH vitamin D, is converted from 25-hydroxy (OH) vitamin D by the kidneys; it is short-lived and thus not a good way to measure body levels, so ask for a 25-OH vitamin D level instead. We get vitamin D from diet and sunlight. A normal 25-OH vitamin D level is considered >30 mg/ml. Anyone with an autoimmune disease should strive for a 25-OH vitamin D level between 55 and 70 mg/ml. This includes patients with inflammatory bowel disease (such as Crohn's disease or ulcerative colitis). Always check your levels three months after starting a supplement to assess your response.

10. **Trace Minerals.** These include zinc, selenium, and magnesium. The best way to measure how much of the mineral you are actually retaining is by checking a red blood cell level. If your levels are low, first try to increase natural dietary sources. I prefer the food-based route here and consider supplements only if the levels are markedly low or you are showing signs of mineral deficiency.

Using the approach in *Happy Gut* and the Gut C.A.R.E. Program, even the sickest person has a template for recovery from the worst of gut imbalances. The functional tests I describe in this chapter will help you uncover those imbalances. Once you complete the Happy Gut Diet and Gut C.A.R.E. Program, if you still have lingering symptoms, the tests in this chapter are part of your road map back to health. They are meant to help you uncover the root causes.

Lynne, age sixty, felt her health was very good, although she was experiencing slightly elevated blood pressure. She asked her doctor to run my "Ten Common and Not-So-Common Tests Everyone Should Have" as part of her annual physical. Although Lynne's diet included a minimum of processed foods and added sugar, the test results indicated she had deficiencies in vitamin D, omega-3, and magnesium as well as a thyroid imbalance, an elevated fasting glucose level, and high triglycerides. Armed with this information, she immediately eliminated bread and other hidden sources of sugar from her diet and saw a marked improvement in her blood pressure. As an added bonus, she lost five pounds in the first two weeks.

By finding what's out of balance, we merely have to give the body the right nutrients, targeted supplements, sometimes anti-yeast and anti-parasitic herbs, and the right setting (mental, spiritual, and physical) to restore it back to a state of optimal health.

A GUIDE TO TESTING BASED ON YOUR SYMPTOMS AND CONDITIONS

Asthma, Allergies, Eczema, Hives	
Tests to Consider:	Celiac workup
	Comprehensive stool analysis
	Delayed food sensitivity testing
	Intestinal permeability assessment
	Small intestine bacterial overgrowth breath test
Therapeutic Interventions:	Happy Gut Diet
	Hypoallergenic protein powder
	Omega-3 supplementation
	Quercetin (500 milligrams twice a day)
	Vitamin C (1,500 milligrams twice a day)
	N-acetylcysteine (500 milligrams twice a day)
Autoimmune Disease	
Tests to Consider:	Celiac workup
	Comprehensive stool analysis
	Delayed food sensitivity testing
	Intestinal permeability assessment
	Methylation defect genetics

Therapeutic Interventions:	Happy Gut Diet (*also excluding nightshades*) Hypoallergenic protein powder Omega-3 supplementation B-complex N-acetylcysteine (500 milligrams twice a day)
Bloating/Excessive Gas	
Tests to Consider:	Comprehensive stool analysis Small intestine bacterial overgrowth breath test Lactose intolerance breath test FODMAP intolerance Delayed food sensitivity testing Celiac workup
Therapeutic Interventions:	Happy Gut Diet Low FODMAP diet Anti-*Candida* diet Digestive enzymes Berberine (500 milligrams twice a day) Oregano oil (500 milligrams twice a day) *Candida* control supplements Hypoallergenic protein powder L-glutamine
Chronic Diarrhea/Loose Stools/Post-Infectious "IBS" (after a "food poisoning")	
Tests to Consider:	Celiac workup Comprehensive stool analysis Comprehensive parasitology profile Fecal fat analysis Lactose intolerance breath test Fructose intolerance breath test FODMAP intolerance
Therapeutic Interventions:	Happy Gut Diet Hypoallergenic protein powder Low FODMAP diet *Saccharomyces boulardii* (10 billion CFUs every four to six hours until resolved) Probiotics

Constipation	
Test to Consider:	Comprehensive stool analysis
	Fasting glucose (to rule out diabetes)
	Delayed food sensitivity testing
	Celiac workup
	Colonoscopy
	Thyroid function tests
Therapeutic Interventions:	Cultured foods
	Omega-3 (1,000 milligrams twice a day with food)
	Probiotics (30 billion–100 billion CFUs)
	Magnesium citrate (starting at 200 milligrams at bedtime)
	Aloe vera
	Triphala

Fatigue	
Tests to Consider:	Celiac workup
	Comprehensive stool analysis
	Delayed food sensitivity testing
	Intestinal permeability assessment
	Methylation defect genetics
	Saliva cortisol/DHEA profile
	Urine organic acids
Therapeutic Interventions:	Happy Gut Diet (*also excluding nightshades*)
	Hypoallergenic protein powder
	B-complex
	Herbal adaptogens (ashwagandha, ginseng, rhodiola)
	N-acetylcysteine (500 milligrams twice a day)
	Omega-3 supplementation
	Probiotics
	S-acetyl glutathione (200 milligrams two to three times a day)

Fibromyalgia/Generalized Muscle Pain	
Tests to Consider:	Celiac workup
	Comprehensive stool analysis
	Delayed food sensitivity testing
	Intestinal permeability assessment
	Methylation defect genetics
	Urine organic acids

Therapeutic Interventions:	Happy Gut Diet (*also excluding nightshades*)
	Hypoallergenic protein powder
	B-complex
	Curcumin (500 milligrams twice a day)
	Magnesium glycinate (200–400 milligrams three times a day)
	N-acetylcysteine (500 milligrams twice a day)
	Omega-3 supplementation
	Probiotics
	S-acetyl glutathione (200 milligrams two to three times a day)
	**Fullness Immediately After Eating**
Tests to Consider:	Fasting blood glucose
	Gastric emptying scan
	Low stomach acid (trial of betaine HCl)
	Small intestine bacterial overgrowth breath test
Therapeutic Interventions:	Aromatic or Swedish bitters
	Digestive enzymes/betaine-HCL
	Frequent, small meals
	Berberine (500 milligrams twice a day)
	Happy Gut Diet
	**Inflammatory Bowel Disease**
Tests to Consider:	Celiac workup
	Colonoscopy and/or endoscopy
	Comprehensive stool analysis
	Comprehensive parasitology profile
Therapeutic Interventions:	Digestive enzymes
	Happy Gut Diet/Specific Carbohydrate Diet[2]
	High-potency probiotics (for example, VSL#3)
	**Irritable Bowel Syndrome**
Tests to Consider:	Comprehensive stool analysis
	Small intestine bacterial overgrowth breath test
	Lactose intolerance breath test
	FODMAP intolerance
	Delayed food sensitivity testing
	Celiac workup

Therapeutic Interventions:	Happy Gut Diet/Low FODMAP diet
	Digestive enzymes
	Hypoallergenic protein powder
	Probiotics
	Prebiotic foods
	L-glutamine

Leaky Gut Syndrome	
Tests to Consider:	Comprehensive stool analysis
	Delayed food sensitivity testing
	Celiac workup
	Intestinal permeability assessment
Therapeutic Interventions:	Hypoallergenic protein powder
	L-glutamine
	DGL
	Aloe vera
	Zinc carnosine

Migraines	
Tests to Consider:	Comprehensive stool analysis
	Delayed food sensitivity testing
	Celiac workup
	Intestinal permeability assessment
	Urine organic acids
Therapeutic Interventions:	Happy Gut Diet
	Omega-3 (1,500 milligrams twice a day)
	Butterbur (500 milligrams twice a day)
	Riboflavin, a.k.a. vitamin B_2 (50 milligrams daily)
	Magnesium glycinate (200 milligrams twice a day)
	Sleep hygiene
	Stress reduction

Nutrient/Vitamin Deficiencies	
Tests to Consider:	Small intestine bacterial overgrowth breath test
	Blood tests: vitamins B_{12}, folic acid, B_6; D 25-OH; iron; ferritin; CBC; homocysteine; red blood cell zinc/selenium/magnesium; NutrEval
	Urine organic acids

Therapeutic Interventions:	B-complex
	Hypoallergenic protein powder
	Targeted supplementation
	Trace mineral supplementation

Sour Stomach/Acid Reflux	
Tests to Consider:	Endoscopy
	H. pylori antibodies and stool antigen
	Comprehensive stool analysis
Therapeutic Interventions:	Chewable DGL before each meal
	Aloe vera
	Zinc carnosine
	Frequent, small meals
	Probiotics
	Treatment for *H. pylori* if present

Yeast Overgrowth	
Tests to Consider:	Comprehensive stool analysis
	Stool DNA PCR
	Urine organic acids
Therapeutic Interventions:	Happy Gut Diet/Candida Diet
	Berberine (500 milligrams twice a day)
	Oregano oil (2 to 3 drops four times a day)
	Herbal anti-*Candida* supplements
	Antifungal medications
	Digestive enzymes
	Probiotics

LOOKING FOR ROOT CAUSES

Let's look at all the ways your gut may become dysfunctional. We will start by focusing on food reactions in more detail, then move on to diagnosing specific types of conditions. For more information on the types of tests you can run to uncover your gut imbalances, visit www.happygutlife.com.

FOOD INTOLERANCES, ALLERGIES, AND SENSITIVITIES

There are two main types of food reactions. One is an immediate reaction, mediated by immunoglobulin E (IgE) antibodies, and the other is a delayed food reaction also known as a delayed sensitivity, mediated by immunoglobulin G (IgG) antibodies. Not all food reactions are immune mediated.

Food Intolerances

Remember, a food intolerance (like lactose intolerance) is not a food allergy. An intolerance results from a digestive enzyme deficiency, which makes it difficult to break down a certain food nutrient. The intolerance symptoms are experienced as:

- Gas
- Bloating
- Indigestion
- Abdominal cramping or pain
- Flatulence
- Often loose stools or diarrhea

Food Allergies

We also need to distinguish a food allergy from a food sensitivity. What we understand as a food allergy is known as a type 1 hypersensitivity reaction, which is IgE mediated, like the reaction people may get to a bee sting if they are allergic. It causes an *immediate* response that can begin within seconds to minutes after contact with the substance. The characteristics of a food allergy may include:

- Skin rash (redness or flushing)
- Hives
- Itching of the skin or throat
- Anaphylaxis
- Shortness of breath or an asthma attack

Understanding food allergy testing:

Our immune system has different protective mechanisms, just like a country's defensive forces are divided into land, air, and sea, so while one test may be negative you can still have a reaction to a given food via another mechanism.

Our antibody defenses are split up between A's, E's, G's, and M's. I test for IgE antibodies to foods only when an immediate reaction occurs to rule out an allergy to the specific food. The most common IgE-triggered food allergies are to peanuts, pine nuts, and shellfish.

EOSINOPHILIC ESOPHAGITIS:
AN UNUSUAL TYPE OF FOOD ALLERGY

Another type of food allergy, which is becoming increasingly common, is caused by *eosinophils,* a special line of white blood cells that are mobilized in allergic responses. Eosinophils invade the esophagus and cause inflammation there, leading to a condition known as eosinophilic esophagitis. It presents with episodes of sudden, alarming chest pain when swallowing food. It can feel like the food gets stuck in the middle of the chest while traveling down. It is diagnosed by a procedure called an endoscopy. The best holistic treatments for this condition are to remove high-sensitivity foods from your diet and to chew your food well.

Food Sensitivities

The other type of reaction to food is known as a sensitivity. This involves a prolonged or delayed reaction to the food substance, and it is facilitated by a different type of antibody, known as IgG.[3] People are often shocked when they are told a food they commonly eat and consider to be healthy may be at the root of their problems. Unlike IgE-mediated food allergy, the response is not immediate.

The symptoms and characteristics of IgG food reactions include:

- Delayed onset (several hours up to thirty-six hours after the exposure)
- Hives (may also occur)
- Skin rashes (like eczema)
- Fatigue
- Mental fog
- Asthma
- Irritable bowel syndrome
- Migraines[4]

Because these responses are delayed, the problem-causing foods are notoriously difficult to identify.

Diagnosing food sensitivities:

Food sensitivities are what I am most concerned with when testing for food reactions. As we previously discussed, IgG antibodies can have widespread effects throughout the body in sites far from the gut, which makes them great masqueraders.

The best way to tell if you are food sensitive or intolerant is to keep track of your symptoms and then eliminate that specific food as part of the Happy Gut Diet (discussed in Chapter 2) while logging how you feel in the food and symptom diary (Appendix B).

How to test for food sensitivities:

Two testing protocols are generally used by laboratories to identify food reactions: the radioallergosorbent (RAST) assay and the enzyme-linked immunosorbent assay (ELISA). RAST is used to identify immediate (IgE-mediated) sensitivities, and ELISA (IgG) is used to identify both immediate and delayed food sensitivities. Neither test is perfect, but the ELISA is more precise in identifying specific IgG antibodies to foods.

Generally, all reactions should be avoided, but depending on lifestyle and practical matters, you can eliminate the foods to which you have the severest reactions first and then move on to less severe ones as you get used to the changes in the way you are eating.

LEAKY GUT SYNDROME

Gut "hyperpermeability," or leaky gut syndrome, was once something that only alternative medicine practitioners talked about. Recent research, however, is elucidating the underlying mechanisms and proving to mainstream medicine that this syndrome actually exists. As discussed in Chapter 1, leaky gut syndrome explains the underlying pathology in many of the gut-associated diseases we are working to reverse. The symptoms of a leaky gut overlap with those caused by food sensitivity reactions.

Diagnosing Leaky Gut Syndrome

There is no perfect test for leaky gut syndrome. As is often the case in medicine, the diagnosis is based on the impression of the health-care practitioner and grounded in a thorough history of your symptoms. If a food sensitivity blood panel shows a multitude of moderate to severe reactions, you can be sure that underlying these reactions is a leaky gut. The most objective measure, however, is a positive intestinal permeability test.

If you have a leaky gut, the Gut C.A.R.E. Program is designed to heal the gut lining and return intestinal permeability to normal. Along with completing this program, I encourage you to work with a Functional Medicine practitioner to uncover the root causes of your leaky gut, like hidden food sensitivities. The Gut C.A.R.E. Program and Happy Gut Diet will address most of these issues; however, you may require an additional individualized approach to fix your unique imbalances.

GLUTEN INTOLERANCE VS. CELIAC DISEASE

As previously discussed, gluten intolerance or sensitivity is one of the biggest links between inflammation in the gut and systemic disease. Gluten sensitivity and celiac disease (which are perhaps all part of one big spectrum) may be characterized by:

- Acid reflux
- Bloating
- Abdominal pain
- Distension
- Diarrhea
- Difficulty gaining weight (or alternatively, weight gain)
- Constipation

What we have learned in the last fifteen years is that celiac disease can also lead to all sorts of conditions, like:

- Iron-deficiency anemia
- Rashes (like dermatitis herpetiformis or hives)
- Type 1 diabetes
- Migraines
- Autoimmune thyroid disease
- Sjögren's syndrome (an autoimmune disorder)
- Ankylosing spondylitis
- Rheumatoid arthritis[5]

This is why celiac disease has been called the "great modern-day imposter." You do not need to have gut symptoms to have celiac-associated conditions.

HOW CELIAC DISEASE DESTROYS YOUR GUT AND YOUR HEALTH

The small intestine villi are tiny, fingerlike projections (almost like a shaggy carpet) that allow for the greatest amount of absorption. When a person develops celiac disease, the villous lining of the small intestine (often called a brush border because it looks like the bristles of a brush) suffers from the inflammation and is flattened out. This reduces the total area available to absorb nutrients and leads to vitamin and mineral deficiencies.

Diagnosing Celiac Disease

Dr. Alessio Fasano, an expert in celiac disease, has recommended a better way to diagnose celiac disease or gluten sensitivity.[6] When four of the five factors below are present, the diagnosis of celiac disease is confirmed:

1. Symptoms of celiac (digestive, allergic, autoimmune disease, inflammatory disease)
2. Elevated antibodies to gluten (antigliadin [AGA] or tissue transglutaminase [tTG] antibodies)
3. Positive small intestinal biopsy
4. Improvement of symptoms on a gluten-free diet
5. Genetic markers for gluten sensitivity are present (HLA-DQ2 and -DQ8)

How to Test for Celiac Disease

Note that when checking for blood markers for celiac disease, you may test negative if you happen to be IgA deficient (that is, your body makes less IgA immunoglobulins) even if you in fact have celiac disease. So whenever these tests are run, a baseline IgA antibody level should also be checked.

1. **Tissue transglutaminase (tTG) IgA antibody:** A highly sensitive test for celiac disease. It is one of four criteria proposed by Dr. Fasano to diagnose celiac disease. By itself, it is not conclusive, but is highly suggestive. A negative test rules out the disease 98 percent of the time.
2. **Deamidated antigliadin IgA/IgG:** A newer test now used predominantly for celiac disease because it has a higher level of accuracy than the prior antigliadin antibody (AGA) test. If total IgA levels are low (as in an IgA-deficient person), then the deamidated

AGA-IgG level can help diagnose celiac disease even in this setting where the other antibodies will be negative.

3. **Antigliadin antibody (AGA) IgA/IgG:** The older test for diagnosing celiac disease, but it may also be positive in individuals with gluten sensitivity. It is not as accurate as the newer deamidated antigliadin antibody tests.

DIAGNOSTIC CRITERIA FOR GLUTEN SENSITIVITY*

1. When you eat gluten, you get immediate digestive or body symptoms (like migraines, headaches, nasal congestion).
2. After a period of avoidance, when you reintroduce gluten into your diet, the same symptoms occur.
3. Typical allergy tests for IgE to gluten and/or wheat and skin prick testing are negative.
4. Antigliadin antibodies (of the IgG class) may be positive (approximately 50 percent of the cases).
5. Other celiac disease tests are negative.

*I believe the *first two* criteria alone are enough to diagnose gluten sensitivity. The other criteria merely support the diagnosis and help differentiate it from celiac disease.

LACTOSE INTOLERANCE VS. DAIRY SENSITIVITY

Many people with IBS suffer from a lactose intolerance. When they remove dairy from their diet, they immediately feel better simply because they've reduced their exposure to lactose.

A dairy sensitivity results from an immune reaction to one of two main dairy proteins: casein or whey. Immune reactions can develop in the form of antibodies (IgG, IgA, or IgE) or as cellular immunity (in sensitized individuals, white blood cells release destructive and inflammatory granules like hand grenades when exposed to dairy proteins). Any single mechanism or combination of these can lead to a dairy sensitivity. The possible symptoms of a dairy sensitivity are the same as any other food sensitivity.

Diagnosing Lactose Intolerance vs. Dairy Sensitivity

The easiest way to test for lactose intolerance is to remove lactose (dairy) from the diet and observe for improvements in your abdominal symptoms (a reduction in gas, bloating, and distension) and even in the consistency of your stool (more solid and formed and less diarrhea). If you have IBS, you should eliminate dairy. This does not necessarily have to be for a lifetime, but for some, long-term avoidance will result in the greatest gut happiness.

How to Test for Lactose Intolerance

Another way to evaluate if lactose specifically is contributing to your gut symptoms is to use a diagnostic breath test, which is very safe and noninvasive. A positive test shows an increase in the levels of hydrogen in your exhaled air, confirming the fermentation of lactose by gut bacteria. This test could raise your blood sugar, so if you are diabetic or insulin resistant, it should be done under the guidance and supervision of a health professional.

How to Test for Dairy Sensitivity

The best way to tell if you are dairy sensitive is to keep track of your symptoms while eating dairy, then eliminate dairy as part of the Happy Gut Diet while logging how you feel in the food and symptom diary. When you get to the Reintroduction Phase for dairy, pay close attention to any symptoms (no matter how small they may appear) after you consume anything containing dairy.

To test for dairy sensitivity, which involves the immune system, we check for antibodies. IgG, IgE, or IgA antibody (immunoglobulin) levels to dairy proteins (casein, whey) can be measured in a blood test. You will find recommended laboratories for this type of testing in Appendix D.

INTOLERANCE TO FODMAPS

FODMAPs stands for "fermentable oligo-, di-, and monosaccharides and polyols (sugar alcohols)." What makes these compounds in food so problematic is that they attract water, are not easy to digest, are poorly absorbed (unless cleaved by enzymes), and are rapidly fermented by gut bacteria, which leads to increased water and gas in the gut.

High-FODMAP foods contain:

- Lactose
- Fructose
- Fructans
- Galactans
- Sugar alcohols (polyols)

The symptoms of FODMAP intolerance mimic the symptoms of IBS and other gastrointestinal disorders. These symptoms include:

- Abdominal pain or cramping
- Gas
- Burping
- Bloating
- Flatulence
- Constipation and/or diarrhea

A low-FODMAP diet has been clinically and scientifically proven to reduce abdominal symptoms in people suffering from irritable bowel syndrome, celiac disease (not responding to a gluten-free lifestyle), and inflammatory bowel disease (in remission, with low inflammation). The Happy Gut Diet limits these foods, but you should be aware of each one of the FODMAP components so that you can make any slight alterations in your diet to improve your gut symptoms.

Lactose:

See page 160 for a full discussion of lactose intolerance. Note that in addition to cow's milk, lactose is also found in sheep's and goat's milk. Symptoms usually occur within thirty minutes to two hours after consuming dairy products.

Fructose:

Fructose is a carbohydrate found in fruit, honey, maple syrup, agave syrup, and, of course, high-fructose corn syrup (HFCS). Foods high in fructose, such as red apples, pears, and mangos, are more likely to trigger symptoms.

Fructans:

Fructans are short-chain carbohydrates containing a chain of fructose molecules. They are sometimes referred to as fructooligosaccharides (FOS), a common prebiotic found in artichokes, leeks, garlic, onions, and jicama. (For more on prebiotics, see Chapter 3.)

The highest intake of fructans in people's diets worldwide comes from wheat. Since we lack the enzyme to break down fructans, eating too much often leads to bloating, gas, and pain. If you overdo supplementation with prebiotics (such as FOS powder), though, you may develop these symptoms as well.

Galactans:

We also lack the enzyme to break down galactans. The foods highest in galactans are beans and lentils.

Polyols:

Sugar alcohols is another name for polyols. They are naturally found in some fruits and vegetables, but more often they are found as added sweeteners in sugar-free gums, mints, cough drops, and medications. Limit the following sugar alcohols:

- Sorbitol
- Mannitol
- Maltitol
- Erythritol (the least likely to cause gut distress)
- Xylitol (also found in toothpastes and Xlear Nasal Spray, a natural, nonsteroidal sinus decongestant)

Many people suffer from unrecognized sensitivity to polyols but fail to make the connection when they are chewing gum, for example. Symptoms can be quite subtle, so really tune in to your body to notice them.

For a more detailed guide, including which foods are high and low in FODMAPs, visit www.happygutlife.com.

Diagnosing a FODMAP Intolerance

If you have a FODMAP issue, avoiding high-FODMAP foods will lead to a reduction in your bloating, discomfort, gas, abdominal pain, and diarrhea. As you avoid these foods, there will be fewer short-chain carbohydrates in your diet for the bacteria in your gut to ferment.

How to Test for a FODMAP Intolerance

If your symptoms are so pervasive that it is hard to notice differences immediately with dietary changes, then a diagnostic breath test can help determine what is causing your underlying symptoms.

YOU'VE GOT A PARTY GOING ON IN THERE: BACTERIA, YEAST, AND PARASITES

When your gut ecosystem shifts from a predominance of friendly to a preponderance of unfriendly bacteria, yeast, or parasites, the resulting microbial imbalances can wreak havoc in your digestive tract, including dysbiosis, small intestine bacterial overgrowth, and yeast overgrowth.

These are not conditions that traditional Western medical tests are adept at detecting and treating. The specialty labs in Appendix D provide enhanced testing methods, which expand the diagnostic capabilities of health-care practitioners.

DYSBIOSIS

One of the most common disorders of the gastrointestinal tract is a dysbiosis. When you have a dysbiosis, the predators in your internal garden have taken over and are throwing an unwelcome party in your gut. If symbiosis means "living in harmony with," then dysbiosis is the opposite—"living out of harmony with." In dysbiosis, the delicately orchestrated ecosystem inside your gut has lost its state of harmony with the rest of your body.

Even though we generally think of the gut when we talk about dysbiosis, it can occur on any mucosal or barrier surface in the body—the respiratory tract, sinuses, nose, lungs, ears, nails, skin, and vagina. Unlike food poisoning or traveler's diarrhea (which is also a form of abrupt dysbiosis), the type of dysbiosis we are looking for is usually subtle. It evolves over time and can exist in the background for months or years as it wreaks all sorts of havoc around your body. For example, if you are a woman with recurrent vaginal yeast infections, you can be certain that your gut microbiota is harboring an overgrowth of yeast and losing favorable bacteria.

Dysbiosis also represents a dysfunctional response between a host (your gut and body) and a microbe. Patients with autoimmune or inflammatory conditions may have a misguided immune response to a friendly microbe. These microbes tend to live in their own symbiotic, protective colonies within biofilms. A biofilm is a slimy coating that surrounds the microbes like a shield, protecting them from the body's defense mechanisms and also serving as a way to trap and share nutrients. Biofilms can become particularly problematic in chronic infections because our immune system cannot penetrate it. Specific herbs or other probiotic bacteria are often necessary to break through the biofilm shield.

Causes of Dysbiosis

The number one cause of dysbiosis is **antibiotics**. Whether you've been on antibiotics once in your lifetime, once a year, or once every few months, this exposure has disrupted the natural floral balance in your gut. Other common causes include:

- Chronic indigestion or acid reflux (especially when it leads to the use of an acid-reducing drug, like a PPI)
- Chronic constipation (slow transit allows for organisms to grow out of balance)
- Stress (suppresses healthy levels of *Lactobacilli* and *Bifidobacteria* and reduces the secretion of protective IgA antibodies)

The symptoms of dysbiosis are nonspecific and are seen in a variety of conditions. You may have a dysbiosis if you suffer from recurrent:

- Diarrhea
- Constipation
- Gas
- Bloating
- Indigestion
- Feeling of excessive fullness after meals

Extraintestinal (outside of your gut) symptoms of dysbiosis may include:

- Rashes
- Hives
- Eczema
- Asthma
- Nerve pain or numbness in your hands and feet
- Joint swelling (such as an inflammatory arthritis)

Diagnosing Dysbiosis

The internal environment of the digestive system must be analyzed to diagnose dysbiosis. This can be done directly through the analysis of a stool specimen or indirectly through analysis of metabolites detected in the urine. Each of these tests has its own strengths and weaknesses.

Stool studies:

Stool studies are an essential and obligatory part of a gut analysis. These can be subdivided by the methods used in the stool analysis as follows:

1. **Detection of undigested food particles:** The presence of meat and vegetable fibers in the stool reveals digestive enzyme deficiency.

2. **Detection of fecal fats:** Fecal fat, triglyceride, and cholesterol measurements show how well fats are being absorbed. As a result, if fecal fat is elevated, fat-soluble vitamins may be deficient because of malabsorption. If triglycerides are elevated, you may be suffering from pancreatic insufficiency, low stomach acid, or insufficient bile production. If cholesterol is high, you may have malabsorption or SIBO (see next section).

3. **Markers of digestion:** Detecting fecal fat, triglycerides, cholesterol, and meat and vegetable fibers are indirect markers of digestive function.

4. **Metabolic analysis:** There are several measures of healthy bacterial metabolism in the gut:

• **Short-chain fatty acids (SCFAs)** are an indirect measure of the adequacy of dietary fiber and prebiotic foods that help feed the gut flora. The right amount of SCFAs are necessary for the health of the colon.

• **N-butyrate** is a marker of the energy supply for the colonocytes (the cells that line the colon). Colonocytes preferentially use butyrate for their energy needs, so an adequate amount of butyrate from colon bacteria helps keep your colon healthy.

• **Beta-glucuronidase** is an enzyme produced by anaerobic bacteria (those that live without oxygen) in the gut that cleaves bile, allowing bile to be reabsorbed into the body from the intestines. This is important because glucuronidation is one of the most important Phase II liver detoxification pathways for the excretion of carcinogens, toxins, and steroid hormones. The liver, through a series of reactions, anchors (or conjugates) a toxin or steroid hormone to glucuronic acid and then excretes the complex into the bile for elimination in the intestines. Waiting there are these renegade bacteria that, with their beta-glucuronidase enzyme, break the anchoring bond to glucuronic acid. The toxins and hormones are reactivated and reabsorbed into the body, where they continue to cause damage or hormone excess.

5. Measurement of Inflammatory Markers:

a. **Eosinophil protein X** (EPX) is one of several major inflammatory proteins secreted by eosinophils (the same white blood cells involved in eosinophilic esophagitis). The level of EPX in the stool is a marker for inflammation, even at low levels. The following conditions are associated with a high fecal EPX:

- Inflammatory bowel disease
- Intestinal parasites (like helminthiasis)
- Chronic diarrhea
- Food allergies or sensitivities
- Celiac disease
- Allergic colitis
- Acid reflux

b. **Calprotectin** is a protein mainly produced and released by neutrophils (a type of white blood cell) in response to mucosal damage. It has an ability equivalent to antibiotics to kill both bacteria and fungi. It is an extremely stable protein, unchanged by medications, dietary supplements, or enzymes. It can be found in stool for more than seven days after an inflammatory event and can also predict relapses in IBD. An elevated calprotectin is found in IBD, but not IBS.

c. **Lactoferrin** is a glycoprotein also secreted by neutrophils, and like calprotectin, it has antimicrobial properties. It is another marker for inflammatory activity in the gut but is not as sensitive as EPX and calprotectin for detecting low levels of inflammation.

6. **Stool culture for bacteria and yeast:** A culture plate is used to grow bacteria and yeast from the stool sample. To increase the yield of this test, normally three separate stool specimens are requested. The downside of this method is that it is not always easy to grow every organism present in the GI tract. The upside is that when an organism is cultured, you can be sure it is present, and it can be tested for its susceptibility to antimicrobials. Beneficial, along with potential pathogenic, bacteria and yeast may be discovered using this method.

7. **Stool DNA by PCR analysis:** This is a controversial method that is capable of detecting minute amounts of the DNA of bacteria, yeast, and parasites in the stool. Organisms that are typically very difficult to grow in culture, such as anaerobic bacteria, can be detected using this method. The downside of this method is that it is not clear whether DNA fragments actually represent the active presence of the organism.

8. **Microscopic exam for parasites and worms:** A microscope is used to examine a representative sample of the stool submitted to the lab to determine the presence of parasites or worms.

9. **Detection of parasite antigens:** This is usually via an ELISA (enzyme-linked immunosorbent assay), a type of immune test that detects protein molecules unique to certain parasites (like *Giardia lamblia*, *Cryptosporidium*, and *Entamoeba histolytica*). If the parasite is present in the stool specimen, this test will be positive.

10. **Detection of *Clostridium difficile* (*C. diff.*) toxins A and B:**
This bacteria causes severe diarrhea that can eventually lead to so much inflammation that the colon enlarges and becomes immobile. Most harmful strains of *C. diff.* secrete toxins A and B, which are responsible for the diarrhea and inflammation by irritating the cells that line the intestines. Toxins A and B are measured by an ELISA, a highly sensitive test, and are either positive (present) or negative (not present).

Urine organic acids testing:

Organic acids are weak acidic compounds produced by metabolic processes, either our own or our microbial inhabitants. Microbial organic acids are produced through fermentation. Unique organic acids produced by different bacteria and yeast give them an identifying signature. People with chronic illnesses, including neurological and mental disorders, often are found to excrete elevated levels of several abnormal organic acids. This is due to an overgrowth of bad microorganisms in their guts, resulting in a wide variety of symptoms from mood and movement disorders to hyperactivity, fatigue, and immunological dysfunction.

SIBO (SMALL INTESTINE BACTERIAL OVERGROWTH)

SIBO is a type of **dysbiosis.** It stands for small intestine bacterial overgrowth (sometimes also called BOSI—letters scrambled, same acronym—or SBBOS [small bowel bacterial overgrowth syndrome]). It is estimated that 50 to 75 percent of patients with IBS have SIBO (diagnosed by a hydrogen breath test) and benefit from treatments to reduce SIBO.[7] Unlike the large intestine, which is teaming with microorganisms, the small bowel often has less than 10^4 organisms per milliliter.[8] SIBO is caused by an overpopulation of bacteria in the small intestine that normally do not form part of its balanced ecosystem. It can also result from an over-predominance of generally friendly bacteria, which leads to increased fermentation of the sugars in the carbohydrates you eat.[9]

The symptoms of SIBO overlap with many other disorders, but the most salient of them is an inability to tolerate the simple carbohydrates in starches, sweets, sugars, and fibers, or even supplementation with a probiotic, without developing uncomfortable symptoms of:

• Gas
• Bloating
• Distended abdomen within fifteen minutes and up to three
  hours after a meal

But may also include:

• Flatulence
• Nausea
• Vomiting
• Diarrhea (including steatorrhea or greasy, loose stools because
  of fat malabsorption)
• Fatigue
• Signs of malnutrition and malabsorption (including weight
  loss and vitamin or mineral deficiencies)
• Weight gain (paradoxically) from fluid retention and
  inflammation[10]

If you have any of these symptoms or if you have recently taken or currently take an acid reducer, such as a PPI (like Nexium, Aciphex, Protonix, or Prilosec) or H_2 blocker medication (like Pepcid or Zantac), and experience any of these symptoms, you should get tested for SIBO.

Malnutrition because of SIBO results from overpopulated bacteria consuming nutrients before they can be absorbed. These bacteria also inflame your small bowel, which reduces the absorption of nutrients. In conjunction with having abdominal symptoms, you may also feel weak and fatigued.

You will notice there is some overlap between the symptoms of SIBO and symptoms of yeast overgrowth (see the next section). The self-test for yeast overgrowth will help you better distinguish if your symptoms are more likely yeast related.

Diagnosing SIBO

There is no perfect test for diagnosing SIBO, and often my colleagues treat presumptive SIBO based on symptoms but not on objective data. The best times to test are when symptoms are vague, the person does not respond to conventional therapy, or, as in cases of presumed SIBO, the symptoms mimic other root causes, such as yeast overgrowth.

How to Test for SIBO

1. **Small bowel aspiration:** The gold standard for diagnosing bacterial overgrowth in the small bowel is an aspirate from the jejunum or middle portion.
2. **Hydrogen and/or methane breath test:** This is the best noninvasive test to diagnose small intestine bacterial overgrowth. The test is based on the fact that there are no other sources of hydrogen or methane production in humans. After a twelve-hour overnight fast, a baseline breath sample is taken, then at various time intervals after a sugary drink breath samples are taken.
3. **D-xylose breath test:** Similar to the hydrogen/methane breath test, a D-xylose breath test uses a 25-gram drink of the sugar xylose.

The methods are similar to the other breath test; however, this test increases the ability to detect SIBO from 60 to 90 percent.[11]

CANDIDIASIS/YEAST OVERGROWTH

Yeast overgrowth and candidiasis (excessive presence of *Candida sp.*, an unfriendly yeast, in the gut) are forms of a yeast-predominant dysbiosis. Your best protection against this is a normal acidic stomach pH, but any acid-blocking medication or infection that makes your stomach less acidic may lead to yeast overgrowth. Once established, yeast overgrowth and the toxins produced by them will wreak havoc throughout your body, leading to a host of seemingly unrelated symptoms and conditions.

When I talk about yeast overgrowth, I need to make a distinction between what this is and the classic form of yeast infection or widespread candidiasis seen in immunocompromised individuals. The type of yeast overgrowth seen most commonly in non-immunocompromised patients is an ecological imbalance in their GI tracts (and in women, intravaginally as well). In these cases, *Candida* has become a predator, wiping out other friendly, symbiotic bacteria. A diet rich in sugar and simple carbohydrates is the culprit.

COMMON SYMPTOMS OF YEAST OVERGROWTH

- Fatigue
- Poor memory, mental fog
- Insomnia or excessive need for sleep
- Anxiety
- Mood swings
- Muscle and joint pains
- Alcohol intolerance
- Itching or rashes

- Excessive bloating, especially after meals (and almost to the point of looking pregnant)
- Cravings (sugar and starchy foods)
- Abdominal pain

Diagnosing Yeast Overgrowth or Candidiasis

The diagnosis of yeast overgrowth or candidiasis is often inferred from symptoms and clinical judgment. The self-test on page 176 is a good way to figure out if you may have problems with yeast. There are also objective tests that are not perfect but can aid in the diagnosis when symptoms are too vague or could be caused by more than one source (as is often the case).

How to Test for Yeast Overgrowth or Candidiasis

1. **Stool testing via microscopy and culture:** Specialty labs (see Appendix D: Resources) can analyze stool for the presence of yeast.
2. **Serum testing:** Just like for food sensitivities, you can be tested for IgG, IgM, and IgA antibodies to *Candida*. *Candida* immune complexes—basically antibody molecules that are stuck together by *Candida* antigens (proteins) into complexes of two or more—may also be detected.
3. *Candida* **DNA by PCR (polymerase chain reaction):** This is a very sensitive test for the presence of up to five different species of *Candida* in the bloodstream. It is used to test for candidiasis but also shows promise in detecting more indolent overgrowth in the guts of persons suffering from yeast dysbiosis.

4. **Stool PCR testing:** This test uses DNA amplification to identify microorganisms in the gut, including *Candida* and anaerobic bacteria that were previously very difficult to isolate in culture.

5. **Microbial organic acids testing:** D-arabinitol is a metabolite of the five-carbon sugar arabinose that can be detected in the urine. *Candida* species produce arabitol, which is absorbed and then converted to arabinose by the liver. The kidney secretes the final metabolite, which when high is very suggestive of yeast overgrowth in the GI tract.

Take the following test to assess whether you suffer from yeast over-growth.

SELF-TEST FOR YEAST OVERGROWTH

Question	Yes	No
1. Have you taken antibiotics repeatedly (<4 weeks each time) or for prolonged courses (>4 weeks)?	4	0
2. Do you feel tired, achy, and a general malaise?	4	0
3. Do you suffer from PMS, menstrual irregularities, mood swings, and/or sexual dysfunction?	4	0
4. Have you been bothered by recurrent vaginal yeast or prostate infections or urinary discomfort?	3	0
Have such infections been severe or persistent?	1	0
5. Have you had chronic athlete's foot, ringworm, "jock itch," or other chronic fungal infections of the skin or nails?	3	0
Have such infections been severe or persistent?	1	0

6. Are you unusually sensitive to strong chemical odors, smoke, perfumes, and colognes?   2   0

7. Do you suffer from poor memory or an inability to concentrate? Do you feel "spaced out" at times?   2   0

8. Have you taken prolonged courses of prednisone or other steroids? Have you taken birth control pills for >2 years?   2   0

9. Do sweets and simple carbs seem to trigger your symptoms?   2   0

10. Do you crave sugar?   1   0

11. Do you suffer from constipation, diarrhea, bloating, abdominal pain, or distension?   1   0

12. Does your skin itch, tingle, or burn? Are you troubled by unexplained rashes?   1   0

13. Do you see a white coating on your tongue?   1   0

Your Total Score = _____

INTERPRETING YOUR RESULTS:

Add up your total score. Add an extra point for severe or persistent infections in questions 4 and 5. Interpret your results below based on your gender.

- A score of 12 or greater for women/10 or greater for men suggests that your health problems may be connected to yeast overgrowth.
- A score of 16 or greater for women/14 or greater for men indicates that your symptoms are most certainly yeast related.
- A score of 20 or greater for women/18 or greater for men means you have severe yeast problems.

FUNCTIONAL GUT IMBALANCES

Functional gut imbalances are disruptions in how the gut performs its daily functions. This may be a reduced ability to make acid, enzymes, or digestive juices, or a disruption in the ability of the gut to act as a barrier to large food particles and unfriendly organisms.

ACID REFLUX/INDIGESTION

If you are like the millions of people around the world who suffer from acid indigestion, heartburn, excessive burping, gas, bloating in your upper abdomen soon after you eat, or nausea before or after meals, you have a stomach acid imbalance. Before you turn to medication, you need to look at your diet and lifestyle. Diet often plays the primary role. Secondarily, acid reflux is a mechanical issue, as the pressure from too much food, incompletely digested and sitting in the stomach, especially at bedtime, pushes stomach acid up past the lower esophageal (LE) sphincter, which protects the bottom of the esophagus. This leads to pain, inflammation, and a burning sensation in your chest.

Medications that suppress stomach acid may make your immediate symptoms better, but they should never be part of a long-term strategy to manage your reflux or indigestion. I am not against achieving immediate relief when it is needed through OTC or prescription drugs, but ultimately acid reflux is a diet and lifestyle issue. Staying on these medications for extended periods of time may have dangerous, long-term health effects.

If you suffer from symptoms of hyperacidity or reflux, you first need to rule out an infection with *Helicobacter pylori*.

H. PYLORI INFECTION

Your doctor may suspect a *Helicobacter pylori* (*H. pylori*) infection if you have symptoms of a stomach ulcer. It is one of the most common chronic bacterial pathogens affecting people worldwide. Symptoms may include:

- Nausea
- Vomiting
- Lots of belching
- Indigestion
- Abdominal pain in the upper abdomen

H. pylori is transmitted orally through kissing or even the sharing of cups or utensils. It is unique in that it can live in the unfriendly acidic environment of the stomach. Within the mucosal layer of the stomach, it raises the pH (making it less acidic) to protect itself by producing ammonia.

If left untreated, *H. pylori* can cause inflammation or irritation of your stomach lining (known as gastritis) and even lead to ulcers in the stomach or duodenum. It also provokes an immune response in the gastric-associated lymphatic system that at its worst can lead to MALT (mucosa-associated lymphoid tissue) lymphoma, a type of stomach tumor.

How to Test for *H. pylori* Infection

A variety of tests detect *H. pylori* and can help determine whether you have an active infection; here are the most common:

Blood tests (show exposure but cannot determine active infection):

1. **H. pylori IgG antibody levels:** This is the type of antibody that develops within two to four weeks following an infection and is responsible for long-term immunity against a virus or bacteria.
2. **H. pylori IgM antibody levels:** IgM antibodies arise within two weeks of a new infection and can often be used to diagnose a new infection when IgMs are present (and IgGs are absent) because they tend to disappear over time. However, in some people IgMs will linger longer, so they are best used as a screen for the further testing discussed next.

Tests that show current active infection:

1. **Urea breath test (UBT):** This is an indirect test done by breathing into a special breath collection bag. A baseline breath sample is first collected. Fifteen minutes after drinking a solution of urea, a second sample is collected. If there is an increase in the amount of carbon dioxide exhaled, an active infection is verified. The UBT is FDA-approved to diagnose active infection and confirm cure after the treatment of *H. pylori* infection.

2. ***H. pylori* stool antigen (HpSAg):** Antigens or protein particles associated with the *H. pylori* bacteria that trigger an immune response can be measured from a stool sample. This test is highly sensitive, making it a great noninvasive test for active infection. It is also FDA approved to monitor the response to therapy and afterward for a cure.

3. **Endoscopic biopsy:** A gastroenterologist can perform an endoscopy to diagnose *H. pylori* via a tissue sample of the stomach. This is used to diagnose active infection and to confirm cure; however, it is invasive, and other tests are less invasive, less expensive, and just as sensitive.

If you have active infection with *H. pylori*, you may be treated with very powerful antibiotics and acid suppressors. They will result in a dysbiosis, even if one did not exist prior to the therapy. The potency of the antibiotics is hard on the digestive system, and often people struggle to make it through the two weeks of therapy.

There are also natural therapies that may be used to eradicate *H. pylori*, but the treatment time will be much longer. Regardless of the eradication method, before and after *H. pylori* eradication therapy you should follow the Gut C.A.R.E. Program protocol to restore your gut's ecosystem.

LOW STOMACH ACID

Low stomach acid often masquerades as acid reflux after eating. Yes, you read that correctly. It's a paradox. On the one hand, stomach acid *is* reaching unprotected areas of the esophagus, causing the burning feelings associated with hyperacidity. However, with low stomach acid, food sits undigested in the stomach longer, which increases the likelihood that pressure inside your abdomen will push the food upward. To make this paradox worse, medications that lower stomach acid production seem to make it better, but they are not correcting the real problem, which is acid reflux.

COMMON SIGNS AND SYMPTOMS OF LOW STOMACH ACID

- Bloating, burning, and gas in the upper abdomen immediately after meals
- Dilated blood vessels in the nose or cheeks (a.k.a. rosacea)
- Nausea after taking supplements
- Multiple food allergies
- A sense of "fullness" immediately after eating that does not go away
- Undigested food in your bowel movements
- Rectal itching (also a sign of yeast overgrowth)

Self-Test for Low Stomach Acid

The most common sign of low stomach acid is a feeling of bloating or stomach expansion *immediately* after eating a protein-rich meal or within the first thirty minutes. If you experience this on a regular basis, you most likely have low stomach acid and would benefit from supplementation.

A basic test for stomach acid insufficiency is to take a hydrochloric acid supplement (known as *betaine hydrochloride*) during a protein-rich meal and see how it makes you feel. Start with 650 milligrams of betaine hydrochloride during a meal or immediately after (within thirty minutes of finishing the meal). If you feel *no* discomfort (pain, nausea, or a slight burning sensation) after taking the hydrochloric acid replacement, then your stomach is *not* producing enough acid, and you need to supplement with it. At every third protein-rich meal use one more capsule to a max of five capsules or until a sensation of warmth occurs in your stomach. A warm feeling means you have surpassed your max dose, so cut back by one capsule at the next meal and so on until no discomfort occurs once more. The right dose will help you digest proteins better without causing any discomfort.

If you continue to feel discomfort, there may be an area of inflammation, and you should consult with your doctor.

DIGESTIVE ENZYME DEFICIENCIES

Digestive enzymes break down the foods we eat into absorbable units that can be utilized by our bodies. Total body wellness depends on the proper breakdown and assimilation of nutrients from our foods. Digestive enzyme deficiencies have a variety of causes, including:

• Stress
• Malnutrition
• Toxicity (exposure to environmental toxins)
• Imbalanced stomach pH
• Inhibitors in food (lectins and phytates—antinutrients that are discussed in Chapter 2)
• Infection/inflammation (anywhere in the gut or the organs of digestion)
• Free radical damage from eating inflammatory foods
• Removal of the gallbladder (results in bile salt insufficiency)

The symptoms of digestive enzyme insufficiency are extensive when you take into account all of their downstream effects. If you cannot digest your food properly, you will suffer from nutrient deficiencies, abdominal distress, dysbiosis, and protein malnutrition. Your potential to develop leaky gut syndrome and food sensitivities is high, along with all the symptoms associated with these conditions. The diagnosis of digestive enzyme deficiency is usually based on symptoms and your response to enzymes, rather than testing. If your symptoms improve with a digestive enzyme supplement, then it is assumed that you had a deficiency to begin with.

- Fullness lasting two to four hours after a meal
- Bloating, gas, and flatulence occurring one to three hours after a meal
- Presence of undigested food in your stool
- Weight loss or weight gain (malnutrition occurs with both calorie underconsumption and overconsumption)
- Clay-colored, fatty stools (steatorrhea) resulting from the inability to split and assimilate dietary fats; also may be due to a bile salt insufficiency
- Deficiency of fat-soluble vitamins, such as A and K, because of fat malabsorption, leading to fatigue and general malaise

PANCREATIC ENZYME INSUFFICIENCY

The pancreas produces very important digestive enzymes that help you break down proteins and fat. A deficiency in these enzymes often leads to the poor absorption of fats.

Symptoms following a fatty meal will include:

- Bloating
- Indigestion
- Abdominal and/or back pain
- Abdominal distension
- Light-colored stools that float in the toilet bowl

Because the symptoms of pancreatic enzyme insufficiency overlap with other conditions and the deficiency usually occurs in the setting of other gut problems, testing for pancreatic function is helpful for determining whether this is a contributor to your symptoms.

How to Test for Pancreatic Enzyme Insufficiency

A safe and easy self-test is to take a pancreatic enzyme supplement during a fatty meal; if you were deficient, you will not experience your usual symptoms and your stool will be more solid and brown.

Objective markers of pancreatic function, such as *chymotrypsin* and *pancreatic elastase-1,* may also be measured as part of a stool analysis. The levels detected indicate whether there is enough pancreatic enzyme secretion to support healthy digestion. **Chymotrypsin** is a digestive enzyme secreted with the pancreatic juice in the duodenum, where it helps complete the digestion of proteins that was begun in the stomach. **Pancreatic elastase-1 (PE1)** is the best marker for pancreatic function in the stool. It is a protease enzyme, meaning that it helps break down and digest protein. Because it does not break down as it travels down the GI tract, it is an excellent test for pancreatic function.

If you have pancreatic insufficiency, you can improve your symptoms immediately with a pancreatic enzyme supplement. However, since pancreatic insufficiency does not happen in isolation, ask for other tests to look for leaky gut, celiac disease, SIBO, and/or a parasite if your levels are low.

MEDICATION-INDUCED GI DISTRESS

We often create or exacerbate gut distress by taking medications for other issues. We assume that if something is a medicine, it will help us feel better or get well without untoward side effects, but even OTC medications can have serious potential secondary effects. See Appendix E for a list of medications and their potential gut-associated side effects.

The functional tests for gut function are varied and complex. My hope is that after reading this chapter about the underlying causes of gut-related disorders, you'll consider how your diet and gut ecosystem imbalances may be at the root of your chronic condition(s). The Happy Gut Diet and the Gut C.A.R.E. Program have been designed to address the majority of these issues, but the duration and type of therapy (including herbal supplements) can be individualized for you using these functional tests. Use this chapter as a guide to fall back on when asking your doctor for these life-saving tests.

PART IV

A HAPPY GUT, HAPPY LIFE

THE EMOTIONAL GUT: THE MIND-GUT CONNECTION

Nothing could be more critical than getting the word out about the connection between seemingly invisible gluten sensitivity and brain dysfunction.

—DR. DAVID PERLMUTTER, *GRAIN BRAIN*

Y OUR GUT AFFECTS NOT only how your body feels, but it can also affect how you feel in your *mind*. It can be the source of immense suffering and, at the same time, the key to incredible wellness. Not only does treating gut imbalances hold promise for resolving pain, inflammation, fatigue, allergic diseases, autoimmune diseases, and weight gain, but it also offers relief from brain-related disorders—from autism, attention deficit hyperactivity disorder, obsessive-compulsive disorder, and depression to dementia and even Parkinson's disease.

In fact, the gut is often referred to as the "second brain," and for good reason. Remarkable discoveries are showing how your gut can affect your mood and the way your brain functions. Even more surprising is how this is actually a two-way street; researchers have found that the brain also talks to the gut. This conversation offers new ways to think about brain disorders and how to treat them via gut rebalancing. By creating a happy gut through the Gut C.A.R.E. Program, you are simultaneously creating a happy mind and a happy life.

WHO IS REALLY IN CHARGE? YOUR MIND OR YOUR GUT?

There is a two-lane superhighway network of communication between your gut and your brain. Just like the brain has its own nervous system (the *central nervous system,* or CNS), the gut has the *enteric nervous system* (ENS). Both nervous systems actually originate from the same embryonic cells, and this is important because parts of the body that originate from the same embryonic tissue share a synchrony throughout your life in the way they are affected and affect each other.

The enteric nervous system, acting independently from the brain, has a number of very important functions:

1. It coordinates the contraction of the muscle cells that line the intestines to keep everything moving in the right direction.
2. It triggers the coordinated release of gut hormones and enzymes to promote proper digestion as food arrives.
3. It helps open up the circulation to the gut after you eat so the body assimilates nutrients better.
4. It controls the gut-associated lymphatic (immune) system.

All of these functions happen in the background and are communicated to the brain through the *autonomic nervous system.* The two can operate separately and independently, but at the same time they depend on each other, like different branches of the government.

How does this two-way communication affect us? You can have a "nervous" stomach because of thoughts and feelings coming from your mind. However, did you ever consider that you could have a "nervous" (or hyperactive, depressed, demented, or autistic) mind because of trouble arising in your gut? Specifically, this refers to problems such as food sensitivities, an overactive gut-associated immune system, dysbiosis, leaky gut syndrome, small intestine bacterial overgrowth, low stomach acid, yeast overgrowth, and gut inflammation.

Over the years, I have noted how gut imbalances trigger behavioral, emotional, and psychiatric symptoms. Often people are so toxic that it is a struggle to get them to make changes that will improve their health; these changes require drastic modifications in their lifestyle and eating habits. Jamie was one such case.

Twenty-one-year-old Jamie was brought in to see me because he couldn't put on weight and was having behavioral issues. He was anxious, suffered from insomnia, and was underweight. His parents were present at the interview, and although Jamie was already an adult, he mostly allowed his parents to answer for him; he chimed in with little bits of information in short sentences only when I directly asked him a question. His diet included fast food, processed foods, and lots of sugar, bread, pasta, and dairy. While we were in the exam room, I noted that Jamie acted nervously and could not sit still—he constantly fidgeted and moved his legs.

When presented with psychiatric and behavioral disturbances, one of the first places to look is the gut. *Jamie's stool studies showed a dysbiosis with yeast overgrowth, and food sensitivity testing confirmed what I already suspected—a sensitivity to wheat/gluten and dairy, among other foods. Jamie was willing to make small changes in his diet, and we started him on an anti-yeast protocol, which included reducing his sugar intake and taking a daily probiotic supplement. We also agreed that he would first eliminate dairy, which he felt would be the easiest to do.*

When Jamie returned one month later, he appeared to be a different person. He had successfully avoided dairy and drastically reduced his sugar intake for one month. He was less fidgety, and he spoke for himself, noting that he was sleeping better and that his anxiety was markedly reduced (without antianxiety medication, mind you).

As it was for Jamie, an important realization is that you are much more in control of how you feel by how you eat than you realize. At first,

Jamie was resigned to living his life in constant discomfort, but now he had new hope that he could feel normal. As a result, he was inspired to start exercising as well.

Transforming the Mind Through the Gut

Jamie is only one among hundreds of patients I have seen undergo a remarkable transformation in mental symptoms after rebalancing their gut ecosystems. Sadly, often doctors blame psychiatric problems for a patient's gut-related symptoms. The patient-centered approach of Functional Medicine, however, shows that these "psychosomatic" illnesses have real root causes that are being missed in the Western paradigm. My patients' transformations are a testament to the intimate connection between our guts and our brains.

Ultimately, who is in charge? From my experience, it is clear that improving gut health will positively affect brain health. Your gut is talking to your brain, and you control it first and foremost by what you put at the end of your fork.

HOW YOUR GUT RULES YOUR BRAIN

The factors that affect brain health through the gut include:

- Dysbiosis: unfriendly bacteria and/or yeast that produce neurotoxins that slow your ability to think and affect your memory retention.
- All the conditions that lead to a leaky or "hyperpermeable" gut.
- The gut immune response to partially digested food proteins that get through the gut lining, such as gluten, and the effect of gluteomorphins (discussed on page 200) on the brain.
- Chronic gut inflammation, which leads to the release of inflammatory signals from the gut immune system that affect how the brain functions and may also

contribute to depression. This inflammation can actually change the levels of neurotransmitters and increase stress hormone secretion.[1,2]

- A diet too rich in fermentable simple starches, which results in the overgrowth of gut bacterial species that produce gas and toxic ammonia (a neurotoxin that damages brain cells and is usually detoxified by the liver).

So bottom line: when your gut is out of balance, a chain reaction of bacterial/yeast imbalances and immune and neurological events interfere with your brain's ability to do its job. Communication between the two works against you, and the only way to break this vicious cycle is to make the changes in your diet and lifestyle that will result in total body as well as brain wellness. These modifications, along with a well-thought-out supplement and herbal regimen created and supervised by a Functional Medicine practitioner or naturopath, will help give you your health back.

Tuning In to Gut Feelings

The gut is not only the seat of all health, but it is also the seat of our intuition. I'm sure that at many points in your life you have had a *gut feeling* about something—that intuitive sense that you should do something or avoid someone or some event. It's a very visceral response, best felt when in the negative, as in an aversion to something, some person, or some activity that is felt as nausea, indigestion, or an upset stomach. Your gut feelings are often confirmed by what happens in the situation you were concerned about.

Other times your gut is simply registering your excitement or nervousness with a feeling of "butterflies" in the stomach around a situation that will turn out okay in the end (like a big event in your life or a speech).

The brain tries to make sense of it, but in the background is your "second brain" that seems to know before your thoughts are put into words. Young children, who have not evolved the analytical brain to override what they are truly *feeling*, seem particularly adept at this. Children use this sixth sense to guide their responses. As adults, we have to rediscover our ability to let go of the overanalyzing, overthinking mind and trust in the feelings we get about people and situations.

Our gut feelings are the most powerful ally we have to guide us, protect us, and help us navigate through the complexities of life. By learning to listen to your gut, you are steered in the direction of what's right for you, while ignoring those gut feelings often leads to more suffering.

LISTENING TO YOUR GUT

The best ways to develop your ability to listen to your gut feelings are to:

1. **Practice deep listening:** Put all your attention on what is being said by others, both words and body language.
2. **Meditate:** Bring mindfulness into every part of your life.
3. **Learn to trust your inner voice:** Especially when it comes to making food choices.
4. **Breathe:** Use your breath to create inner peace (see Chapter 8).
5. **Find your center in stressful situations:** Use yoga (see Chapter 8) and meditation. We are always ultimately in control of the way we react to any given situation. Take a step back and create distance to foster understanding of what is happening.
6. **Practice acceptance:** Create inner safety by knowing that what you are experiencing is okay and that your gut feelings are here to help you achieve the greater good.

SEROTONIN, THE GUT, AND HAPPINESS

Serotonin, one of the molecules of emotion, is the signal for a "happy mood" in the brain. However, more serotonin receptors are found in the gut than in the brain. In fact, 95 percent of serotonin found in the body is produced by the gut's nervous system. Being in charge of producing so much of this "happy chemical," along with about thirty other neurotransmitters, it's no wonder the gut is central to feeling happy.

Serotonin has been the focus of much research since the discovery of antidepressant medications called selective serotonin reuptake inhibitors (SSRIs), which were initially believed to be the cure for depression. SSRIs increase the amount of serotonin that remains at the connections between nerves available for nerve-to-nerve communication. By using SSRIs, only about 50 percent of participants in clinical trials experienced a reversal of their depression and/or anxiety. But at the same time these medications change brain chemistry, they can wreak havoc in your guts. Alterations in serotonin signaling in the gut may actually either trigger or improve irritable bowel syndrome.

Serotonin, secreted by the enteric nervous system, seems to play an important role in the coordinated movement of food down the gut. Therefore, if the body's ability to digest protein into amino acids (the building blocks of neurotransmitters) and absorb them through the brushlike lining of the small intestine is reduced because of disturbed gut function, then it is possible this will also result in constipation owing to the reduced production of serotonin. Consequently, the brain will also suffer from depression on account of a lack of neurotransmitters. By looking at how different gut and brain functions are interconnected and dependent on each other, we see the importance of a whole-body approach to wellness. Instead of thinking of depression as a serotonin deficiency in the brain, perhaps we should be thinking of depression as just another symptom of gut dysfunction.

Gut Bacteria and Mood

Balanced with the right amount of healthy bacteria, our guts promote happy brains. Disturb that balance and allow the wrong bacteria and yeast to take over, which produce all types of toxins that are absorbed, and you end up with all sorts of behavioral and emotional problems. These toxins from unfavorable bacteria and yeast produce a sort of "autointoxication." Your gut environment literally becomes the source of ongoing toxicity for you. And with the bugs producing these toxins, your brain chemistry is changed for the worse.

Throw in your immune system's response, which includes the secretion of all sorts of inflammatory signals that also affect your brain, and your CNS becomes chronically inflamed along with the rest of your body. This inflammation leads to depression, erratic behavior, and even memory problems.

While in some cases psychological or emotional well-being may benefit from psychotherapy, you cannot work effectively on your brain if you are not promoting an environment that reduces brain inflammation. Your brain will function best when its signals are not jammed by toxins, food allergens, dysbiosis, nutritional deficiencies, and stress. Ultimately, your brain's health is connected to your gut, so to work on the brain you have to start with the gut.

THE GUT, AUTISM SPECTRUM DISORDERS, AND BEHAVIORAL ISSUES IN CHILDREN

Children are probably the most sensitive of all to the ravages of dysbiosis in their guts. A bacterial imbalance will be seen as a change in their behavior or personality. This is partly due to an incompletely evolved blood brain barrier (discussed on page 199), making them more susceptible to toxicity arising from the gut. Not surprisingly, this often follows a course of antibiotics to treat an infection. While working in the best interests of the child, pediatricians and parents may not realize the damage caused by these treatments. The dysbiosis created is characterized by unfriendly bacteria and yeast overgrowth. The child, seemingly all of a sudden, starts getting into trouble at school for his or her behavior, but underlying the problem behavior(s) is a drastic change in the gut microbial flora. Instead, the child is diagnosed as having attention deficit disorder (ADD), attention deficit hyperactivity disorder (ADHD), autism spectrum disorders, or mental health problems. Inevitably, both parent and child suffer as they are shuffled through a medical system that is not designed to look for the root causes.

Studies in children with developmental problems (like autism) have confirmed the presence of toxin-producing bacteria in their guts.[3] As is the case with all diseases, certain children are more susceptible than others because of their genetics, environment, and diets. If they are also eating the Standard American Diet, high in sugar, wheat, and dairy, they are causing even more damage to their gut lining. This perpetuates the problem, continuing to fuel the "fire" in their guts that fuels the "fire" in their brains.

As with any adult sufferer, it's not as simple as saying there is a gut dysbiosis happening in the background for all of these children. A lot of detective work is involved in discovering the specific set of disease conditions and individual triggers creating the mental disturbance. Keep in mind the tests we discussed in Chapter 6.

There is no single "magic bullet" cure for these childhood ailments. As with adults, the multifaceted, holistic approach of the Gut C.A.R.E. Program provides the greatest chance for success with children who have these issues. When problem behaviors first begin to arise, the earlier an intervention is implemented, the greater the promise for a complete remission.

YEAST OVERGROWTH, FOOD CRAVINGS, AND BRAIN HEALTH

As you learned in Chapter 1, antibiotic overuse is the number one cause of yeast (*Candida*) overgrowth in the gut. Anyone who has suffered from *Candida* or yeast overgrowth knows the insatiable cravings it creates for the very foods that are promoting its growth and proliferation. Yeast feeds on simple carbohydrates found in white starches, sugars, fruit, processed foods, juices, and, of course, sweets and desserts. People with yeast overgrowth will crave more of these foods.

Eating high-sugar or sugar-equivalent foods feeds the yeast, leading to the production of neurotoxins that cause fatigue, mental fog, mood swings, headaches, problems with memory retention, poor concentration, inability to focus, insomnia, anxiety, and depression. Yeast overgrowth may also lead to blocked nasal passages, recurrent yeast infections, food and chemical sensitivities, and muscle and joint pains. Usually accompanying this yeast overpopulation is a leaky gut, which allows more of these toxins to enter the body. The yeast cross the gut barrier, causing all sorts of diseases that disguise themselves as chronic fatigue, body pain, and infections; fibromyalgia; and generalized malaise. People who suffer from this bounce from doctor to doctor trying to find a solution, but ultimately the solution is in their guts.

The way to reverse yeast overgrowth is to eat a low-sugar, low-starch diet while taking probiotics and anti-yeast/anti-*Candida* herbal remedies (see Appendix C for suggestions). The Happy Gut Diet and the Gut C.A.R.E. Program are great kick-starters for beating your yeast overgrowth.

Leaky Gut and the Blood Brain Barrier

All the factors that cause damage to the inner lining of the intestines—poor diet, inflammation, medications (like anti-inflammatories and antibiotics), environmental toxins, dysbiosis—lead to a leaky gut. Remember, this inner lining is very thin—only one cell layer thick. So when this layer is damaged, inflammation rapidly spreads through the rest of the body. And since this layer is where much of your digestive enzymes are produced, you cannot digest your food effectively without it. Toxins, foreign material, infectious organisms, and partially digested food particles "leak" into your bloodstream. From there they travel to the barrier between the brain's special circulation and the rest of the body, also known as the blood brain barrier (BBB).

WHAT IS THE BLOOD BRAIN BARRIER?

Much like the gut lining, the BBB is a fine mesh that allows certain substances to get through and keeps others out. This selectivity protects the brain and spinal cord from harmful substances or infections that may have entered the bloodstream. However, the BBB can also be damaged by the same substances it is trying to keep out:

• Environmental toxins
• Medications
• Chronic infections
• Neurotoxins
• Recreational drugs
• Gluten
• Inflammatory foods
• Alcohol

Once the BBB is damaged, it allows these harmful substances to enter the brain and spinal canal, leading to neurological conditions like:

• Depression
• Autism
• Attention deficit disorder (ADD)
• Attention deficit hyperactivity disorder (ADHD)
• Fibromyalgia
• Generalized anxiety
• Chronic neurological diseases
• Chronic pain

It is very common to have a "leaky" brain when you have a "leaky" gut. In Functional Medicine, it is said that "inflammation in the gut equals inflammation in the brain." To heal the critical BBB, you have to address the gut as well by following all the steps of the Gut C.A.R.E. Program in Chapter 3 and using the diagnostic tools in Chapter 6. This includes *at minimum* a gluten-free and dairy-free diet. Also pivotal in restoring the BBB to normalcy is stress management. Later in this chapter and in Chapter 8, we will give you the practical tools for reducing stress in your life through yoga, meditation, and breath work. Finally, supporting neurotransmitter production through a diet rich in whole foods and digestive enzymes and reducing total body inflammation through omega-3 supplementation (especially DHA for the brain) and anti-inflammatory botanicals (like curcumin; see Appendix C) are of utmost importance in restoring brain function.

OPIATES IN YOUR FOOD ARE FOGGING YOUR BRAIN

When a person has a weak digestive system resulting from any of the factors we discussed in Chapter 6, he or she often produces low levels of digestive enzymes. This is particularly problematic when two proteins, gluten (from wheat) and casein (from dairy), are digested poorly. *Gluteomorphins* and *caseomorphins* are formed, and these proteins (products of partial digestion) actually stimulate opium receptors in the brain, leading to all sorts of behavioral and mental problems. They are harmful to your brain and at the root of many mental disorders.

If the gut barrier is also leaky (which is often the case), then the gluteomorphins and caseomorphins easily get into the body and make their way to the brain, where they cause mental fog, short attention spans, attention deficits, and depression and can even aggravate autism spectrum disorders. Since these proteins are detected as "foreign," the body's immune system is also activated, leading to even more problems because of the inflammatory signals that cause the brain to malfunction. These "morphine-like" or "opium-like" gluteomorphins and caseomorphins disturb the brain's performance in the same way these drugs would.

In the Activate portion of the Gut C.A.R.E. Program, using digestive enzyme supplements is an important part of the treatment plan because they help split apart these "toxic" proteins. In doing so, they facilitate your recovery from the inflammation that is plaguing your brain.

MEDITATION AND THE GUT

Stress is a huge factor in how your gut behaves or misbehaves. At the root of stress is the fight-or-flight response—an adaptive reaction that through the ages served to protect us from life-threatening situations. This is a heightened state of response (accompanied by increased heart rate, tense muscles, and hypersensitive skin) that is controlled by stress hormones (such as cortisol and epinephrine). As a sudden reaction that gets you to safety, this response serves its purpose, but over the long term, it results in all sorts of issues, from gut problems to neurological issues, numbness, fatigue, insomnia, and memory problems. For many people this adaptive response is activated for too long without enough of its counterbalancing "relaxation" response.

One way to create this relaxation response is through a mindfulness practice like meditation. Meditation is the most powerful tool for creating a sense of peace within, even when still surrounded by the day-to-day stressors of life. You cannot control what happens outside of you or what happens to you, but you can certainly control your internal state of mind. Ultimately, how you respond to stressful situations is really the only thing that you have control over. Worrying, getting angry, and arguing with others does not change the external events that have transpired. In fact, they damage you by promoting the release of stress hormones and putting you into that fight-or-flight response that sets your entire body, including your immune system and your gut, on high alert.

HOW MEDITATION HELPS WITH GUT HEALTH

Meditation is a form of mindfulness that reduces stress hormones, relaxes the gut, and promotes digestion. In practice, it is a watchful awareness of yourself, and even others, without judgment. Meditation is really about putting aside the ego self and observing yourself with compassionate detachment. What this means in the simplest terms is *breathe*. Yes, the breath is how you access your calm self. By focusing on the breath, you give your wandering mind direction and bring yourself into the present moment. In the present moment, there is no suffering, there is no worry, no frustration, no regrets, and no discomfort because you are only present in that moment for but one second before moving on to the next moment. So much of our lives are spent worrying about the future or the "could-haves" of the past. Meditation takes you out of that stressful state and into a state of peace, acceptance, and gratitude.

As part of the Gut C.A.R.E. Program in Chapter 3, I introduced you to the Happy Gut daily protocol, which includes a five- to ten-minute meditation to kick-start your day. This is a great way to set your intention for the day, become present in your body, and tune in to what is best for you through your gut feelings. By creating a relaxed state within yourself, your gut will benefit from reduced stress hormones, less muscle tension, and important input from the "relaxation" portion of the autonomic nervous system—the parasympathetic nervous system—that allows it to digest and process food with ease. We will guide you on how to meditate in the next chapter as well as share some very useful breathing techniques to aid your mind in achieving a relaxed state.

COMPLEMENTARY MODALITIES AND GUT HEALTH

Complementary modalities, sometimes called alternative treatments, are very useful tools in the management of gut problems. They can help reduce the fight-or-flight response that accompanies feelings of stress, especially disorders like IBS that are so strongly linked to emotions and anxiety.

Here are the complementary modalities for gut health and how they work:

- **Massage therapy:** The healing power of touch is so important in our daily lives. Human touch through massage is one modality that reduces the production of stress hormones and helps relax the muscles, which in turn creates a more relaxed gut. Massage is a great, immediate rebalancer, but if done without working on cleansing the diet, lifestyle, and negative mental thoughts, its effects are short-lived.

- **Neuromuscular release:** A gentle, targeted massage that focuses on releasing tension in the muscles by accessing the nervous system. Its effects have the ability to last longer than a regular massage.

- **Rolfing:** A deeper type of massage focused on release of the connective tissue (known as *fascia*) that surrounds the muscles. The theory is that this connective tissue gets tight like plastic wrap and prevents the muscles from relaxing. Rolfing also has the ability to get into deeper muscles like the diaphragm that control the body's core. Tension in these muscles may result in the buildup of tension in the gut, which leads to digestive problems.

- **Acupuncture:** An ancient Chinese therapy that is more than two thousand years old and uses tiny needles placed in very specific points along "energy meridians" that traverse the body in well-described pathways. Interestingly, some of the meridians have been found to correlate with the patterns of the fascia surrounding the muscles. Inserting these needles in the body releases feel-good chemicals known as *endorphins*. Treating muscle spasms directly by placing needles in these tight muscles, including needling spasms that may occur along the muscles of the abdominal wall in people with ongoing gastrointestinal problems, helps release tension around the gut.

- **Acupressure:** Another form of massage, sometimes called Shiatsu, which like acupuncture is based on the concept that life energy flows through the body through "meridians." Instead of using needles, pressure is applied directly to acupressure points using the hands, elbows, and feet. For someone with an aversion to needles but who would like to experience relaxation benefits similar to acupuncture, this is a great alternative modality.

- **Craniosacral massage:** Based on the premise that the connection between the brain and the sacrum by the steady, easy flow of cerebrospinal fluid through the spinal canal is of vital importance to health, this modality is designed to bring balance to the central nervous system. It is so gentle that it can even be performed on babies. A deep sense of relaxation is created by bringing balance to this system, resulting in better digestion.

- **Chiropractic care:** Believed to restore nervous communication to and from the gut organs by realigning spinal misalignments. It works with the body's innate ability to heal itself. Most of the intestinal nerves are found in the lower part of the spine. By releasing entrapped or pinched nerves, chiropractic care helps support a healthy intestine.

- **Homeopathy:** The active ingredients in homeopathic medicines are micro-doses of plants, animals, and minerals that relieve the same symptoms they cause at full strength (for example, a micro-dose of a coffee bean helps nervousness). Homeopathy may be used to alleviate many gut symptoms, such as bloating, gas, nausea, and digestive cramps, and is a safe alternative for children. Some of my favorite homeopathic remedies for gut health by Boiron, the largest manufacturer of homeopathic products worldwide, are listed in Appendix C.

EVOLVING SCIENCE: YOUR GUT MICROBIOME IS IN CHARGE

As you can see, a confluence of factors affects both gut and brain health. These two "organs" influence each other in both subtle and obvious ways. By reestablishing balance to your gut ecosystem through the Gut C.A.R.E. Program, you inevitably restore balance to how your brain functions.

In the next chapter, we will delve further into this topic by exploring the body-gut connection. You will learn how you can improve your gut health and general wellness through yoga, breathing exercises, affirmations, and meditation. It is full of practical advice that will help bridge the gap between theory and how you can apply this information to create a happy gut for life.

THE PHYSICAL GUT: THE BODY-GUT CONNECTION

Yoga postures . . . help to massage the internal organs and stimulate the digestive activity so that the entire system works more efficiently.

—KRISTA KATROVAS, *SYNC OF HEALTH*

This chapter was written in collaboration with my friends and yoga teachers Paula Tursi and Janet Dailey Butler.* They have put together a series of yoga poses and breathing exercises specifically designed to help you create and nurture a happy gut. But first, Paula explains the importance of tuning in to our bodies, and what she calls our "mammalian nature."**

"In our fast-paced world, we have disconnected from our mammalian nature," Paula explains, "that is, our basic 'animal' or 'instinctual'

---

* Paula Tursi, the founder of Reflections Center for Conscious Living & Yoga in New York City, teaches workshops on yoga and meditation throughout the world. You can find out more about her work on yoga for organ health at http://reflectionsyoga.com. Janet Dailey Butler is a certified reflexologist and yoga teacher who holds kirtans, an ancient participatory chanting experience, in New York City. You can learn more about her and her work with breath and mudras at http://daileyreflexology.com. It is amazing to have them both join me in bringing you this very special chapter on the body-gut connection and how we can improve it.

** Our "mammalian nature" is a concept developed by Paula's teacher Bonnie Bainbridge Cohen, founder of The School for Body-Mind Centering, author, researcher, educator, and therapist, who has been working with movement, touch, and the body-mind relationship for over fifty years.

selves, what we were before we added all the layers of civilization that distanced us from our physical bodies." We have lost our connection with the rhythm of life and with our own internal rhythms. The body-gut connection is about rediscovering this important relationship, which helps create total body wellness. Our bodies need movement to stay healthy. Movement is an essential part of gut health. (I like to use the word "movement" as opposed to "exercise" because movement encompasses a broader array of activities.)

Nothing fills the spirit and lowers stress hormones like taking a walk in a nature preserve and connecting to the natural world, or sitting by the seashore and listening to the sound of crashing waves. We are surrounded by movement in nature, and yet, in this high-speed world, we have become disconnected from ourselves, from our ancestral ways of life, from our own sense of internal movement, and from our gut rhythms.

For many, exercise means going to the gym and running on a treadmill, or spending forty-five minutes on the elliptical. This can feel more like taking medicine than enjoyment. We have a duty to our bodies to move, but it should not feel like a chore. Any way you get your body moving is exercise, whether through taking a dance class, hiking in the wilderness, playing a pickup game of soccer, or swimming in the ocean.

Research has shown time and again that exercise is good for your heart, for building lean muscle, for improving metabolism, and for balancing your mood and stress. However, new science is showing that exercise may also benefit your gut microbiome—that diverse ecosystem living inside you comprising trillions of symbiotic bacteria that help maintain a healthy digestive system.

A study by the University College Cork looked at how gut microbiota may be affected by exercise. A group of professional rugby players was compared with a control group of age- and weight-matched healthy, nonathletic men; their blood was tested for markers of inflammation, and their stool samples underwent genetic testing to detect their levels of microbial diversity. The athletes (as expected) were in better shape than the men in the control group and had lower markers of inflammation, despite an extreme training schedule that resulted in higher levels of creatine kinase (a marker for muscle damage) in their blood.[1]

Most striking was that the rugby players had a gut microbiota that was much more diverse than that of the control group. One particular bacterium, *Akkermansiaceae,* was especially predominant in the athletes. This species has been associated with lower rates of metabolic disease (like metabolic syndrome X, also known as insulin resistance, which was discussed in Chapters 1 and 2) and a lesser tendency toward being overweight. Of course the athletes' diets were slightly different from the nonathletes', especially in terms of protein consumption: 22 percent versus 15 percent of daily calories. This difference in protein consumption may have played a role, but the exercise was also a key factor.

The study of the microbiome is really only in its infancy. As the science highlights, the message is clear: get out there and move your body. Look for ways to make movement (exercise) exciting and enjoyable. Try to mix it up—find variety in the ways that you move. To that end, this chapter will show you how yoga (which comes from the Sanskrit root *yuj,* meaning "to join" or "to unite") can help you connect to your body and gut. Paula and Janet show us how, through yoga, you can experience a different way of moving and relating to your internal organs that will help you tune in to what is good for your gut.

REDISCOVERING YOUR MAMMALIAN NATURE

Paula shares what she has learned through her work: "As we humans have become increasingly more civilized, we have forgotten how to listen to our instinctual self—our mammalian nature—the inner knowing of things that are not learned but are an innate part of us, encoded in our

DNA." Our mammalian nature is to look after the safety and well-being of the self. It tells us who and what to trust, which foods are beneficial and which are not, and how we can best care for our bodies and move through the world. This natural code has become particularly disrupted around our ability to nourish ourselves and move. Commonly, we find ourselves eating impulsively and compulsively—in service of our mind-driven emotions and desires—rather than in the interests of our actual physical needs. Emotional eating and the world of fast-food choices have taken us further away from true nourishment. When we are tuned in and present, when we listen to our gut wisdom, we know exactly how much to eat, which foods will be the most nourishing, and which foods will make us sick.

YOGA AND THE BODY-GUT CONNECTION

Paula believes that as a practice, yoga can help you access your instinctual self. It is about listening and connecting, which we do through the senses. Our senses allow us to *feel* true hunger rather than stress-induced or anxiety-driven "hunger."

Yoga can help you quiet your mind so you can feel and then release the tension stored in your gut and other places in your body. These unconscious tensions, which can become knots (also called trigger points) along the abdominal muscles or a restricted diaphragm that does not allow you to take full, deep breaths, help perpetuate gut issues and other body-wide health problems.

Yoga can help you to connect your mind to your body and your gut. When these three are connected, you awaken a deeper connection to your true self. You stop judging and abusing yourself and begin to honestly care for and respect yourself.

In our modern lives, this mind-body-gut connection is poorly supported. We have lost the family meal, downtime on the weekends, or anything else that once allowed us to slow down, listen, and relate to each other or simply reflect. Instead, we have more ways to keep ourselves preoccupied. Our interconnectedness appears boundless, but our connections at a human level are being challenged. The Internet keeps us connected to an endless world of information, yet technology has complicated our lives. It has expanded the workweek from five to seven days around the clock. We eat on the run or work through lunch, chained to our screens. The mind is ceaselessly engaged while the body is ignored.

Yoga directs us to remember the body and listen to the body's intelligence. Many people do yoga to become more flexible and stronger, but the practice is not meant to be competitive. In yoga, you are *not* meant to compete with others or yourself. You are *not* meant to overcome or master the body. Yoga is intended to be a dialogue with your body.

In our work together, Paula shared with me the importance of asking the body what it needs. She stressed that when you ask your body what it needs, you might hear something different than what your mind expects: "Today I need to be still," or "I need to breathe deeply," or "My liver (in the upper right part of your abdomen) is sore and needs to move," or "My stomach feels acidic, so I need to relax there." If you are listening closely you will notice that your body's responses are continuous. When you check in, you should feel like you are being led by rather than dictating to your body. You should not ignore or overpower any discomfort or resistance you sense. For yoga, you are where you are at the moment, and that's perfect!

Yoga Calms the Nervous System

When you move with this understanding, you turn on the parasympathetic nervous system (PNS), or your calm self, and slowly turn down the sympathetic nervous system (SNS), or your "internal can of Red Bull."

When the PNS is activated through yoga, breathing, and meditation, your stomach, liver, pancreas, and gallbladder secrete acidic and alkaline digestive juices and hormones to promote healthy digestion.

When you eat on the run, or inhale your food at your desk, you are eating with your fight-or-flight response turned on, and blood flow is shunted away from the digestive system. So your gut slows down or comes to a halt. This is useful in an emergency when you need blood circulation and oxygen directed to your arms, legs, and brain for fast action. However, when this fight-or-flight response is prolonged, your abdominal muscles contract and peristalsis (the coordinated, automatic movement of the digestive tract) comes to a halt, resulting in constipation (sometimes alternating with diarrhea), abdominal pain, and a host of gut-related illnesses. Research has shown that this stress response can actually alter the natural balance of healthy bacteria in our guts, causing the gut ecology to shift in favor of a more hostile group of pathogens.

Yoga, meditation, and breathing exercises can help you balance the parasympathetic and sympathetic nervous systems. When you find yourself getting wound up because of stress, you can easily access the PNS through breathing and meditation to return your body to a natural state of balance. Through yoga, you can change your focus toward health and connection and instantly begin the process of healing and disease resolution. This is the mind-body-gut connection we want to create.

Paula teaches that if you skip your yoga or movement practice, you'll notice that not only do you feel less connected to your gut, but you'll start to make poor food choices, and your gut pays the price. I am in full agreement. As a resident-in-training in internal medicine, yoga was my go-to form of exercise to help relieve stress, reconnect with my sore body from nights on call in the hospital, and overcome the fatigue my hectic schedule created. After a yoga class, my body (gut) always craved food that was light and healthy, rich in vegetables and omega-3 fats.

Having a daily (or every other day) practice of meditation and yoga deepens your connection to yourself. The yoga poses and breathing exercises featured in this chapter are all designed to benefit your gut health so you can live with a happy gut. If your schedule is too hectic to even attempt to incorporate yoga into your life, listening and connecting to your gut can be as simple as taking a moment in your busy workday to take three deep breaths while sitting or standing.

STARTING A YOGA PRACTICE FOR A HAPPY GUT

Starting a yoga practice can seem intimidating at first, especially if you have never done yoga before. Starting in a yoga studio or with private lessons with a certified yoga teacher is a great way to begin your practice and avoid injury. Having a certified instructor observe you is important in the beginning phases to help you know if you are moving into, holding, and moving out of poses correctly—that is, in ways that minimize injuries and maximize health benefits. By going to a yoga studio, you can also learn which props will be the most useful for you, such as a yoga strap or blocks. Yoga requires balance and coordination, but the good news is that if you feel you are challenged in these areas, yoga will help you develop better balance and coordination.

In yoga, remember to *only* do what you can physically do and to not push beyond your limits. Whatever your limits are with movement and flexibility, be patient. They will improve with time.

When beginning your yoga practice, wear comfortable, loose-fitting clothing or flexible clothes that have been designed to move with your body. You may want to purchase a yoga mat[2] first, and add other props as you become more familiar with what you need.

When you are ready to incorporate the following seven poses as part of a daily home routine, please do so. It is easy to transition into yogic movement, breathing, and a brief meditation right after you wake up. Engaging in yogic movement early in the morning helps invigorate the circulation throughout your body and gut, preparing you for eating and setting a positive tone for the rest of your day.

If you can get on the mat with the intention of holding one pose for just ten breaths, your practice will quickly grow. And growth won't be because you are supposed to practice, but because it *feels* good. Feeling connected to your body brings real joy, and you'll naturally want more of it.

BEGINNING A YOGA PRACTICE

What you'll need:*

- Yoga mat
- 2 yoga blocks
- Yoga blanket
- Yoga strap

*These items can be purchased at any online yoga accessories store or local sporting goods store. Although not necessary, as you deepen your practice, you may want these to assist the postures. If you're practicing at home, you can use ordinary items such as blankets, pillows, and a large book (as a block) for your practice.

This is how Paula and Janet guided me to begin my yoga practice:

1. **Sit quietly.** Always start your practice by sitting quietly for at least one minute. Doing this lets your whole being know it is time to become centered and to affirm your intention for the practice.
2. **Tap in.** Take a moment to survey your surroundings and yourself within that space. Notice your breath and how and what you are feeling. Tuning in like this will give you a sense of being instead of thinking.
3. **Deepen your breath.** You can use one of the breathing exercises recommended in the breath work section (see page 235) or use your natural breath. Give the breath a rhythm that can pace your practice.

A great starting point is five to ten minutes of yoga and five minutes of meditation (see the next page for a suggested meditation) every morning. This practice will help you transition from sleep to wakefulness. Start each day of the twenty-eight-day Happy Gut Diet with this routine.

Find a quiet place where you can practice your new morning routine. Taking time for yourself first thing in the morning is an important step in the Gut C.A.R.E. Program. It prevents the stress hormone surge that occurs in the morning when you rush out of bed. A relaxed body is a relaxed gut.

YOGA AND A HAPPY GUT: SEVEN DAYS, SEVEN POSES

Your morning routine for the twenty-eight-day Happy Gut Diet will include one yoga pose for each day of the week. It is designed to be easy to include in even the most hectic schedule because it can take as little as ten minutes of your time each morning. <u>Note: you can do each pose more than once—moving in and out of the pose with your breath.</u> Once you get into the habit, you will come to cherish these ten to fifteen minutes of setting your intention for the day and connecting with your body and gut through breathing and movement.

Below are seven poses for seven days, one for each day of the week. Do them in order first, and then feel free to do them in any order you wish or combine a few together in a short sequence. Listen to what your body needs or is asking for on a particular day.

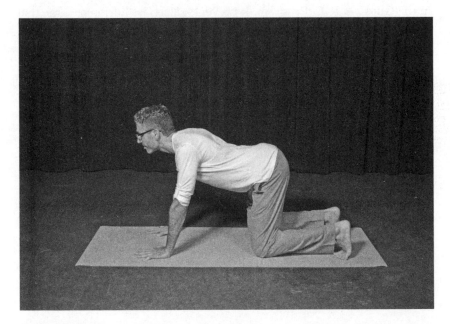

Pose 1a: Cow.

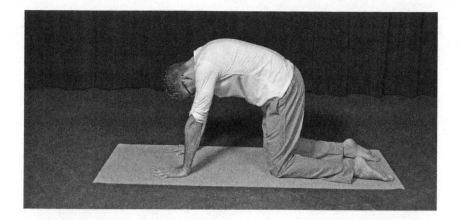

Pose 1b: Cat.

This is a great pose to help you link each breath with your movement and learn to move from your center, where the gut resides, which will move and stimulate the intestines and create circulation around the gut. It is also great for relieving gas and bloating.

1. Start on your hands and knees. Shoulders should be above your hands and knees directly under your hips. Point your fingertips to the top of your mat. Place your shins and knees hip-width apart. Center your head in a neutral position in alignment with your spine, and soften (relax) your gaze downward.
2. Begin by moving into Cow Pose: Inhale as you drop your belly toward the mat. Lift your chin and chest, and gaze up toward the ceiling. Be sure to fully relax your tummy here to give space for your organs.
3. Broaden the area across your shoulder blades and draw your shoulders away from your ears.
4. Next, move into Cat Pose: As you exhale, draw your navel to your spine and round your back toward the ceiling. The pose should look like a cat stretching its back. Here you want to scoop your organs in and up toward your heart.

5. Release the crown of your head toward the floor, but don't force your chin to your chest.
6. Repeat several times. Inhale, coming back into Cow Pose, and then exhale as you return to Cat Pose. Remember to find a rhythm between your breath and the movement.

You can think of this pose as washing your internal body, just like your washing machine washes your clothes.

Cat-Cow Note: This is a very gentle pose, but if you have wrist pain, place your forearms on the floor instead of resting on your hands.

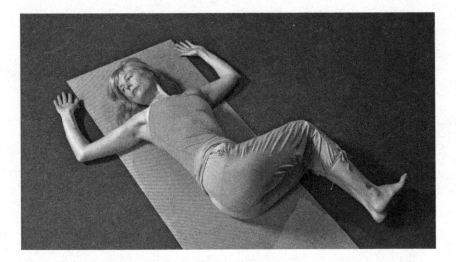

Pose 2: Supine Twist.

This pose gives a much-needed twist to the intestines, which massages your internal organs and tones your abdominal muscles. It is a wonderful pose to promote bowel movements and relieve constipation. It also offers a stretch to the chest and a rotation to the spine, as well as opening up the ribs.

1. To begin, lie on your back with your knees bent and your feet flat on the floor. Let your arms rest at your sides.
2. Exhale and draw both knees to your chest. Spread your arms wide as if you're about to hug someone, or at a right angle as pictured here.
3. Allow your knees to fall to the left while keeping your right shoulder on the floor. At the same time, feel that you can bring the contents of your belly to the right. If your knees don't yet touch the floor you can place a block or a blanket under them for support.
4. Turn your head to the right. Soften your gaze toward your right fingertips. Keep your shoulder blades pressing toward the floor and away from your ears. Allow the force of gravity to drop your knees even closer to the floor.
5. Hold for a few breaths. Exhale and slowly come back to center, bringing both knees to your chest. You can use your arms to hug them closer.
6. Repeat on the opposite side, turning the internal body away from the weight of the knees once again.
7. When you're finished with the pose, hug your knees to your chest for a few breaths, and then slowly exhale as you extend both legs straight along the floor.
8. Be sure to experience the wringing action here. This helps to squeeze the organs in a way that can drain them of old, congested fluid, and upon release this can create a rush of healthier fluid back into the system. Feel free to do this several times.

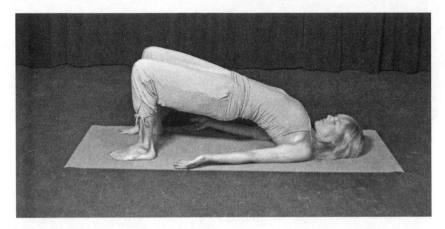

Pose 3: Bridge.

Our third pose works on opening the chest, shoulders, and neck. It also moves the heart and lungs while lengthening the entire line of the gut from mouth to colon. Creating space in the gut line can help soothe and relieve reflux and bloating.

1. Lie on your back with your knees bent forty-five degrees and feet on the floor hip-width apart. Extend your arms along the floor parallel to your body with the palms flat, facing up.
2. Press your feet and arms firmly into the floor. Inhale as you extend your tailbone away from the chest while lifting your hips from the floor.
3. Do not squeeze your glutes; instead, allow them to soften while you draw your navel toward your heart.
4. Roll your shoulders back and underneath your body, squeezing your shoulder blades together to open your heart and lungs. Straighten your arms as much as possible by pressing your forearms into the floor or mat.
5. Keep your thighs and feet parallel—do not roll to the outer edges of your feet or let your knees drop together. Press your weight evenly

across all four corners of both feet. Lengthen your tailbone toward the backs of your knees.

6. Move up and down from this pose, linking the breath and the movement. Inhale to rise and exhale to lower. If you would like to hold this pose, slide a yoga block under the sacrum, just below the lower back. This will help to release tension in the lower back and allow you time to work on opening the chest with deep chest breathing (see chest breath on page 237).

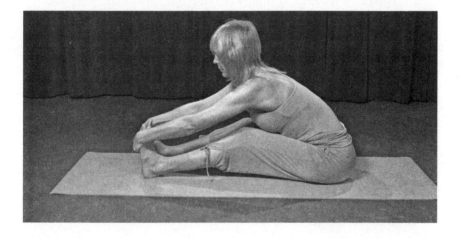

Pose 4: Forward Bend.

Our fourth pose works on stretching the back of the body and compressing the intestine in the lower belly. It is a wonderful pose to stimulate bowel function, relieving bloating, constipation, and reflux, and it creates space for all the organs to flow and function.

Gravity and sitting for long periods of time can cause your torso to compress, which slows down circulation. This pose helps you regain some of that lost space by first compressing and then releasing the lower belly, creating a flush of fluids to a typically stagnant area of the body. It can really help get your bowels moving!

1. Sit on the edge of a firm, folded blanket with your legs extended in front of you. Extend your legs actively as if reaching through your heels. Beginners should bend their knees throughout the pose, eventually straightening the legs as flexibility increases.

2. Inhale while reaching your arms out to the sides, moving in an arc, ending up overhead. Then lengthen your spine and stretch through your torso (gut).

3. While exhaling, bend forward, initiating the movement from the hips and internal organs while keeping your torso long. Keep the front of your torso lengthened. If you are able to, rest your abdomen on your thighs, stretching your chin toward your knees to help keep the front body long and in contact with the legs. This will create the necessary compression of the lower tummy. If not, go as far as you can for now, while not allowing your upper body or chest to collapse when reaching for your toes.

4. Hold on to your shins, ankles, or feet—wherever your flexibility permits. With each inhalation, lengthen the front torso. With each exhalation, fold a bit deeper. Where you are right now is perfect. Breathe.

5. Hold for up to one minute. To release the pose, roll your spine upright one vertebra at a time while supporting with the lower belly.

6. Once you come out of the pose, take a moment to feel the space you have just created in your abdomen.

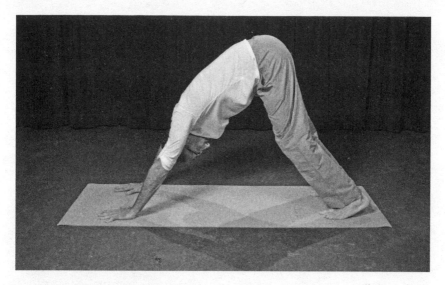

Pose 5: Downward Facing Dog.

Our fifth pose energizes and rejuvenates the body. It can offer a strong stretch to the hamstrings, calves, shoulders, hands, feet, and spine while building strength in your arms, shoulders, and legs. Because your heart is higher than your head in this pose, it is considered a mild inversion. The flow of blood to the brain also calms the nervous system and can relieve feelings of stress that are often the source of gut-related maladies.

Downward Facing Dog is unique because it connects and grounds your entire body. Many gut-related issues stem from feelings of being blocked or stuck both mentally and physically. Downward Facing Dog can give you the much-needed feeling of flow and connection between your body, mind, and gut.

1. Begin on your hands and knees. Align your wrists directly under your shoulders and your knees directly under your hips. The fold of your wrists should be parallel with the top edge of your mat. Point your middle fingers directly to the top edge of your mat.

2. Spread your fingers wide and press firmly through your palms and knuckles. Distribute your weight evenly across your hands.

3. Relax your upper back. Exhale as you tuck your toes and lift your knees off the floor. Reach your sit bones (tailbone) toward the wall behind you as you lengthen the spine. Gently straighten your legs without locking your knees. Pull your hips and thighs away from the shoulders, and keep the extension of your whole body.

4. Firm the muscles of your arms and press your index fingers into the floor.

5. Draw your heels toward the floor by inhaling, then lifting your toes and dropping the heels during the exhale. If you think of this as lengthening through your organs or middle body while using the breath to guide the movement, your heels will naturally reach the floor.

6. Allow your head to hang like a ripe fruit dangling from a tree. Gaze toward your navel.

7. Hold for a few breaths, remembering to keep the spine extended. When you can no longer do this with ease and calm, deep breaths, it is a good time to come out of the pose. Remember to always keep the breath slow and steady.

8. To release, exhale as you gently bend your knees and come back to your hands and knees.

Downward Facing Dog Modification: This is not an easy pose as it requires flexibility in the hips, hamstrings, and shoulders. Feel free to modify the pose by bending your knees more or placing your hands on a chair instead of the floor. Remember its focus is to extend the spine. Do not force the pose.

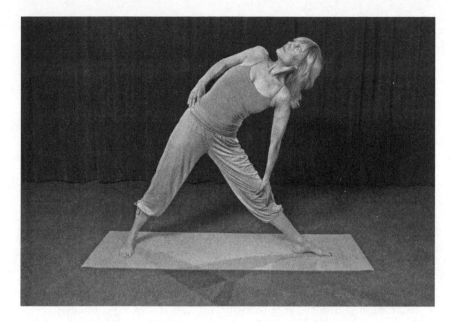

Pose 6: Triangle.

Our sixth pose is a deep stretch for the hamstrings, groins, and hips. It helps relieve lower back pain, and it is an amazing twist for the spine and gut. It stimulates the internal organs, improving metabolism and circulation through the organs of digestion. Whether you are suffering from constipation or intermittent diarrhea from IBS, this pose helps promote balance and calm within the intestines.

1. Stand at the top of your mat with your feet hip-distance apart and your arms at your sides. Feel your breath filling the body from the fingers to the toes. You might imagine yourself as a starfish and send the breath from your center to all six limbs of the body—head and tail included. Take a moment to tune in to your body and draw your awareness inward.

2. When you're ready, place your feet four to five feet apart. Check to ensure that your heels are aligned with each other.

3. Turn your right foot out 90 degrees so your toes are pointing to the top of the mat.

4. Pivot your left foot slightly inward. Your back toes should be at a 45-degree angle.

5. Lift through the arches of your feet while rooting down through your heels and the balls of the feet.

6. Raise your arms to the sides at shoulder height so they're parallel to the floor. Your arms should be aligned directly over your legs. With your palms facing down, reach actively from fingertip to fingertip to open the chest.

7. On an exhalation, reach through your right hand in the same direction as your right foot is pointed. Shift your left hip back so your tailbone and pelvis tilt toward the wall or space behind your left foot. Fold your torso at your right hip. Don't lock your knees.

8. Rest your right hand on your outer shin, ankle, or a yoga block while reaching up as if to touch the sky with your left hand, or alternately rest it on your left hip.

9. Begin to turn the right side of your tummy toward the left, as if you are wringing out your organs. Let the twist originate from twisting your inner body more than from pressing your shoulder back.

10. Draw down through the outer edge of your back foot. Extend equally through both sides of your waist. Lengthen your tailbone toward your back heel.

11. Hold for up to one minute. To release, inhale and press firmly through your feet as you lift your torso. Lower your arms. Turn to the left, reversing the position of your feet, and repeat for the same length of time on the opposite side.

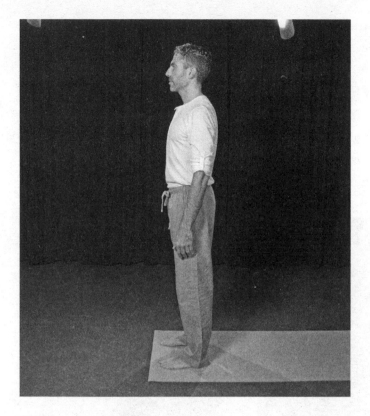

Pose 7a: Sun Salutation.

This is really a series of poses. It's called the Sun Salutation because it can build heat in the inner body just as the sun helps to warm your outer body. It is also done as a way to honor the sun in the sky and the sun as a metaphor for the soul within us. This series of poses is performed in a sequence to create a flow of movements.

Use your breath to guide your movement into and out of each pose. The Sun Salutation is often a warm-up sequence for a yoga practice, but it can certainly stand on its own. It creates a great amount of circulation throughout the body, helping to stimulate a sluggish gut, increase heart rate, and move the lymphatic fluid in the body. (If the Sun Salutation is too difficult for you, Simple Sun, which is easier to start with, can be found on page 234.)

1. **Mountain Pose.** Stand at the front of your mat with your feet hip-width apart and your weight evenly distributed between them, your spine erect, and your arms at your sides. Feel your breath filling the body from the crown of your head to the soles of your feet. Feel yourself as that starfish once more, and send the breath from your center to all six limbs of the body—head and tail included. Take a moment to tune in to your body and draw your awareness inward. Now begin your rhythmic breathing (see page 237).

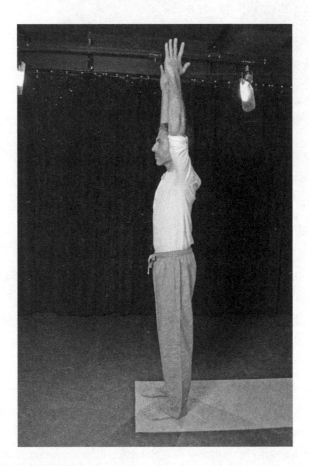

2. **Upward Salute Pose.** Inhale, extending your arms overhead, palms facing each other.

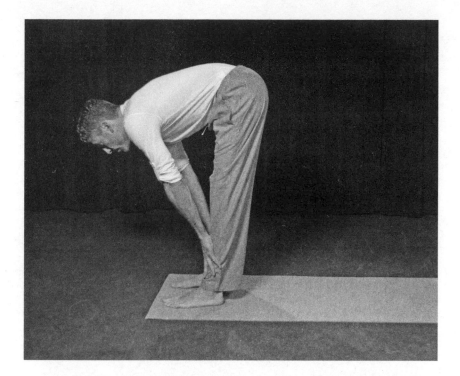

3. **Standing Forward Bend Pose.** Exhale into the Standing Forward
   Bend, bending at the hips and bringing your chest toward your
   thighs and your hands toward the floor. You can bend at the knees to
   make this pose more manageable.

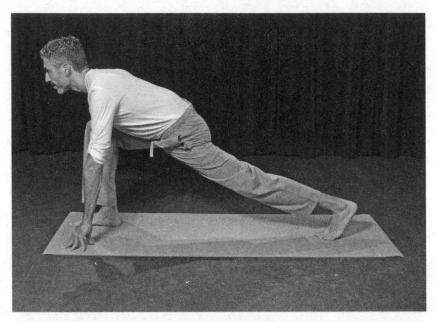

4. **Lunge Pose.** Inhale into the Lunge, placing your hands on the mat
   on either side of your right foot as you lunge your left leg straight
   back behind you. Expand your chest as you lengthen your spine.
   Your right knee should be aligned directly over your heel, not
   beyond, for the safety of your knee.

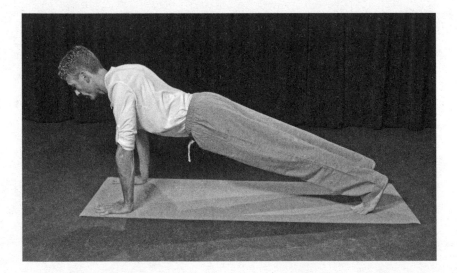

5. **Plank Pose.** Exhale into the Plank, stepping your right leg back so your feet are now side by side. Look straight at the floor, keeping your arms extended and your body straight. Do not lock your elbows. (If you find this challenging to start, rest your knees on the floor.)

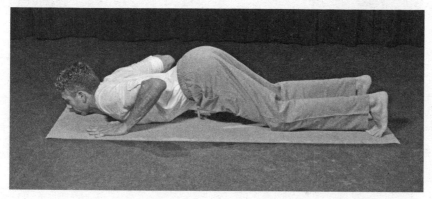

6. **Eight-Point Pose.** Exhale, slowly dropping your knees, chest, and chin to the floor, then let your body and belly rest on the floor. (If you find this too difficult, you can come to all fours and then press your hips back to your heels).

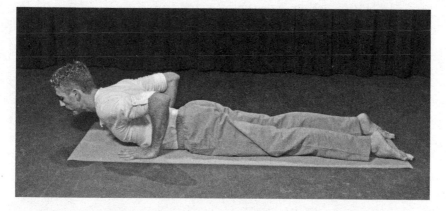

7. **Cobra Pose.** Inhale, pulling with your hands and bringing your chest forward and slightly up off the floor like a cobra. Stretch your legs back toward your feet to avoid pinching your lower back.

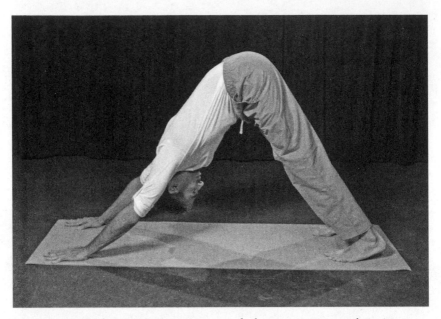

8. **Downward Facing Dog Pose.** Exhale into Downward Facing Dog, tucking your toes and lifting your hips up and back so you're bearing your weight on your hands and the balls of your feet. You did this pose on day five, so it should be familiar. Relax your neck and allow the weight of your head to lengthen your spine. Breathe in and out, lengthening your body and dropping your heels to the floor on the exhale.

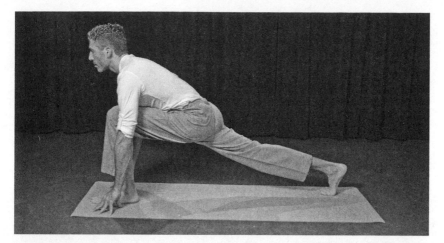

9. **Lunge Pose.** Inhale into the Lunge again, stepping your left foot forward.

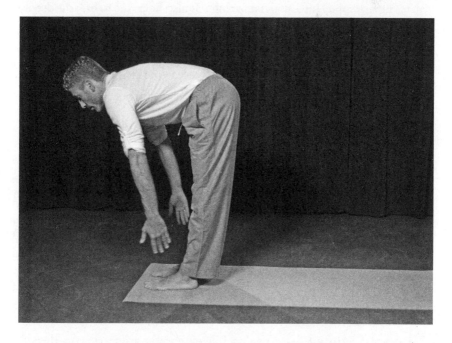

10. **Standing Forward Bend Pose.** Exhale into the Standing Forward Bend again, stepping your right foot forward next to your left foot so your weight is on both feet.

11. **Upward Salute Pose.** Inhale into the Upward Salute again.
12. **Mountain Pose.** Exhale as you bring your arms back down to your sides, completing the Sun Salutation by returning to the Mountain Pose.

Note: You can modify the Sun Salutation series and do it sitting on a chair. Do the parts that you can, if any, off the chair, then return to the chair for the end of the pose.

Pose 7b: Simple Sun.

This is a simple version of the sun salutation that I do every morning. It warms up my spine, hips, and hamstrings. It also helps me to breathe deeply after the shallow breathing of sleep and allows me to welcome the day and get my digestion moving. If you can do only one of the seven poses, make it this series. You will be amazed how it increases your flexibility, builds your breathing capacity, and helps promote bowel movements.

1. **Mountain Pose.** Stand at the front of your mat in the Mountain Pose, with your feet hip-width apart and your weight evenly distributed between them, your spine erect, and your arms at your sides. Feel your breath filling the body from the crown of your head to the soles of your feet. Let go of distractions. Feel yourself as that starfish, and send the breath from your center to all six limbs of the body—head and tail included. Take a moment to tune in to your body and draw your awareness inward. Now begin your rhythmic breathing (see page 237).
2. **Upward Salute Pose.** Inhale while extending your arms overhead, palms facing each other.

3. **Standing Forward Bend Pose.** Exhale as you bend at the hips, bringing your chest toward your thighs and your hands toward the floor. They may likely end up on your knees or shins—that is okay, so don't push or struggle to touch the floor.

4. **Half Standing Forward Bend Pose.** Inhale and bring your hands to your knees or shins and extend your spine. It helps to look ahead of you, which will lengthen the spine away from the hips. Try to keep the legs straight.

5. *Modified* **Standing Forward Bend Pose.** Exhale into the Standing Forward Bend, *but bend your knees,* pressing your belly to your thighs. Then try to line your fingertips up beside your toe tips. It can help to step your feet wider apart to make it easier to touch the floor.

6. **Upward Salute Pose.** Inhale, extending your arms overhead, palms facing each other.

7. **Mountain Pose.** Exhale, completing the Sun Salutation by returning to the Mountain Pose.

BREATH WORK TO HEAL YOUR GUT

Janet explains, "Behind your stomach (in your upper abdomen) is a great network of nerves called the *solar plexus,* also known as the 'seat of your willpower.' It is associated with the power of fire and digestion as well as your 'second brain.'"

Why work with the breath? We all know how to breathe—we wouldn't be alive otherwise—but most of us have periods of time throughout the day or even weeks when we are stressed or worried, and we tighten the chest, keep our bellies in, and feel constricted.

USING THE BREATH TO CREATE SPACE IN YOUR BODY

Try this breathing exercise. Find a comfortable place to sit quietly where you won't be disturbed. Begin to listen to your breath. Don't try to change it, simply listen. How does it sound to you? Is it deep or shallow? Is it comfortable to breathe? Does breathing make your mind calm or anxious? Try not to judge this information. Give yourself the space to be curious about what you feel.

Now let the breath lead you around the body like a guide. Notice what you feel. What part of you moves easily with the breath so that it feels free and open? What part feels sore, agitated, tight, or disconnected? Slowly create movement in the places that feel tight. For example, if a part of your chest wall is not moving, then breathe into it and create more movement there. If a part of your abdomen feels tight, then take your breath there. Listen to your body. Use this exercise to create more space in those areas.

The word "worry" comes from an Anglo-Saxon root meaning "to strangle." Janet explains, "We are literally strangling our life force by holding our breath when we worry, and this restricts blood from flowing freely to our organs. Focusing on the breath is the fastest way that I know to become present and relaxed. When you are truly present, your reactive, worrying mind takes a break."

Four Simple Breaths[3]

These four simple breaths will help clear your mind and promote a healthy gut. All the breath work can be done in a comfortable seated position with the back straight, shoulders relaxed, and belly soft (to allow room for your diaphragm to expand as you inhale), either on the floor with the legs crossed or seated in a chair. You can use these breaths while practicing your daily five-minute meditation.

Rhythmic breath:

1. Open your mouth and make a sound as if you were fogging a pair of glasses.
2. Now make the same sound while inhaling.
3. Repeat a few times. When ready, close your mouth, but continue the breath and sound by lifting the back of your palate while breathing through your nose.
4. Allow a doming (a lifting of the upper palate) in the back of your throat as if you had a mouth filled with marbles.
5. As you progress, let the sound get quieter. You'll hear less sound but you'll feel more sensation.
6. Practice matching the length of your exhalation to the length of your inhalation until there is no separation from one to the other, and it is just one continuous exchange.

   Benefits:
   - Creates heat in the body
   - Soothes and strengthens the nervous system and calms the mind
   - Strengthens the digestive system

Chest breath:

1. Relax your belly and diaphragm.
2. Exhale all the air in your lungs.
3. Keeping the navel close to the spine, inhale into the upper chest.
4. Exhale softly through the lips, continuing to contract the belly.
5. Continue for two to five rounds.

   Benefits:
   - Creates more space between the ribs and in the upper pockets of the chest and lungs

• Promotes healthy elimination

* In a variation, this breath can be done with the arms reaching overhead to help lower anxiety

Three-point breath with Apana mudra[4] (also called a purification mudra):

Note: Do not perform this breath with Apana mudra if you are pregnant.

1. Sit comfortably. Place your hands on the thighs, close to your knees, with palms facing up, and bring the tips of your ring and middle fingers to touch the tips of the thumbs while the other two fingers are stretched out.
2. Begin inhaling through the nose for a count of four, hold the breath for a count of four, and exhale for a count of four.
3. Continue for three to eleven minutes. At the end, inhale deeply, then exhale, and notice how you feel.

   Benefits:
   • Centers the mind
   • Brings your awareness inward
   • Allows you to tune in to your gut feelings
   • Activates the parasympathetic nervous system, creating a general sense of calmness
   • Enhances the eliminative functions of the digestive tract

Long, deep breath:

1. Inhale through the nose, remembering to keep the inhale slow and smooth. Fill the lower, middle, and upper parts of your lungs in that order as the rib cage expands to capacity.

2. Follow with an even, soft, and slow exhale through the nose. This expels all the breath, which empties the lungs while drawing the navel closer in toward the spine.

3. Practice this breath for three minutes. Sit and notice how you feel afterward.

   Benefits:
   - Slows the heart rate
   - Lowers blood pressure
   - Encourages blood flow to the gut
   - Promotes healthy digestion
   - Reduces anxiety and reactivity to stressful situations
   - Helps relax your mind and body
   - Helps bring peace to your mind

Note: The long, deep breath can also be practiced while standing. Use this when you are feeling stressed in the middle of your day. It will bring you out of the fight-or-flight response and back into a more relaxed state.

MAKING TIME FOR HEALING

You may come up against a few obstacles that can derail you from the path to healing your gut, including lack of support and your own beliefs. A huge obstacle we all seem to struggle with is lack of time. Yet making time to care for yourself is essential for real, long-lasting healing.

I'm a big proponent of smaller, more digestible bites. Can you find five minutes for yoga or other movement when you awaken? Can you make time just before each meal to connect and clear your mind? It only takes a few seconds of conscious awareness to make the shift from thinking to feeling. Everyone has a few seconds, right? While a longer practice will increase the magnitude of the health effects on your body and gut, there is no reason you cannot incorporate yoga or any movement practice into your busy life right now.

Your gut health comes down to being in the now—the present moment. Yoga or any movement practice is about the now. It focuses your mind while getting you to stop constantly thinking about the things you worry about. Breathing and movement lower stress hormones, helping to relax your gut. As an added benefit, exercise or simply moving (like going on a hike) is a means to cleanse the mind, body, and spirit.

Let's now make a trip to the Happy Gut Kitchen, where you'll find delicious recipes that will show you how you can make the twenty-eight-day Happy Gut Diet fun and exciting. You won't even miss gluten/wheat, dairy, soy, corn, added sugar, or eggs when you see what a varied menu you can create for your gut cleanse. The meal plan in Chapter 4 shows you how to combine the recipes and make the Gut C.A.R.E. Program an easy transition to a new, healthier, lighter, and more energetic you.

PART V

FUN IN THE KITCHEN

HAPPY GUT RECIPES

WELCOME TO THE HAPPY Gut Kitchen! These recipes will introduce variety to your Happy Gut Diet. The recipes have been created in collaboration with chef Mikaela Reuben (the smoothies and nut milks) and chef and dietitian Marlisa Brown (all the rest) for the Gut C.A.R.E. Program. From unique breakfast smoothies to reinventions of our favorite dishes, we have dreamed up and created recipes that are not only easy on your gut and low in sugar, but also quick and delicious.

By selecting organic (and, when possible, locally sourced) produce, grass-fed beef and lamb, free-range chicken and turkey, fresh or flash-frozen wild cold-water fish, and wild game, you will be eating foods that are healing for your gut and great for your body. With that said, feel free to experiment and make these recipes your own, using ingredients that are local to and seasonal wherever you live.

Be creative, have fun, and come share your creations with the Happy Gut community at www.happygutlife.com.

BREAKFAST SMOOTHIES

Matcha Energizer
Swiss Chard and Strawberry
Raspberry Recharge

Go Green

Spicy Avocado

Blue Ginger

Chocolate-Covered Almond

HOMEMADE NUT MILKS AND DAIRY-FREE KEFIR

Homemade Almond Milk

Coconut-Almond Milk Made from Real Coconut

Coconut-Almond Milk Made from Shredded Coconut

Coconut Water Kefir

SOUPS

Homemade Vegetable Broth

Immune-Boosting Vegetable Soup

Grass-Fed Beef-Bone Broth

Pumpkin Soup with Coconut Cream

Butternut Squash Bisque with Toasted Walnuts

SALADS

Summer Fresh Citrus Salad with Sliced Almonds

Mediterranean Chickpea Salad

Avocado and Organic Heirloom Tomato Salad

Shredded Carrot Salad with Toasted Almonds and Berries

Mixed Greens with Sliced Strawberries

Chicken and Pistachio Lettuce Wraps

Veggie Slaw with Citrus Vinaigrette

Watercress and Jicama Salad

Quinoa Salad with Apples and Walnuts

Dr. Pedre's Scallion Vinaigrette

HEALTHY HOMEMADE SNACKS

Flax Super-Seed Crackers

Nut and Seed Bars

Crispy Kale Chips

SEAFOOD ENTRÉES

Mahi-Mahi with Shallots, Lime, and Veggies in Parchment

Stir-Fried Veggies and Shrimp over Rice Noodles

Roasted Wild Salmon with Dill Sauce

POULTRY ENTRÉES

Roasted Chicken

Chicken Piccata

Stuffed Mexican Turkey Burger

Cilantro Pesto

Chicken Curry

GRASS-FED BEEF AND LAMB ENTRÉES

Beef Kabobs

Bison Burger

Rosemary Lamb

Seared Steak with Dijon-Horseradish Sauce

VEGETARIAN ENTRÉES AND SIDES

Roasted Sweet Potato Wedges with Toasted Pumpkin Seeds

Coconut Brown Rice

Spaghetti Squash with Garlic-Infused Oil and Pine Nuts

Buckwheat Pasta and Vegetables in Homemade Vegetable Broth

Harvest Wild Rice Bowl

Roasted Cauliflower with Toasted Walnuts Topping

Veggie-Stuffed Spring Rolls

DESSERTS

Coconut Macaroons

Almond-Hemp Chocolate Truffles

Fresh Berries with Whipped Coconut Cream

SMOOTHIES

During the twenty-eight-day Happy Gut Diet and Gut C.A.R.E. Program, you will have a carefully crafted smoothie daily for breakfast. The smoothies have been designed to be nutrient-dense meal replacements to start your day off just right.

Feel free to switch out ingredients based on what's fresh, available, and easy to find. For example, you may substitute one green (like Swiss chard) for another green (like organic baby spinach). Or you may want to add flaxseed oil rather than coconut oil. If you are allergic to nuts, then substitute sesame or sunflower seed butter when the recipes call for nut butters. You can alter the recipes to exclude nuts, but note that you may need to use less fluid to adjust the thickness of the smoothie. You may also use ground flax or chia seeds in place of nuts. Experiment, be creative, and share your variations at www.happygutlife.com.

CHOOSING THE RIGHT BLENDER

A high-powered blender is the best choice when making smoothies. I recommend the Vitamix, but you can also use the NutriBullet. This ensures that the nuts, vegetables, and fruit are broken down and well blended together. Older blenders can take a minute or more to get through frozen berries on high, but a Vitamix can do the same

The ingredients are listed in the order in which they should be used. When making a smoothie, blend the mixture as soon as all the ingredients are in the blender. This prevents the protein powder or the nut butter from getting stuck to the bottom of the jar. If you prefer thicker smoothies, then start with less liquid and add more as you desire; if you like your smoothies a little thinner, then continue to add liquid until you have achieved your desired smoothie thickness.

I encourage you to make your own almond milk. Recipes for almond milk and almond-coconut milk are included after the smoothie recipes. Feel free to use either in the smoothie recipes that call for almond milk, or add the almond-coconut milk whenever you would like a little more creaminess in any smoothie.

A few notes on ingredients:

• All the smoothie recipes call for raw cacao powder. Cocoa powder and raw cacao powder are not necessarily the same thing. Raw cacao powder is the raw cacao from the cacao tree without anything else added. In North America, cacao powder is usually processed at high temperatures and then filled with added sugars and milk products and called *cocoa powder.* This is usually the base for hot chocolate. Raw cacao powder is not sweet at all and is much healthier for you, providing trace minerals and antioxidants.

• Coconut butter and coconut oil are both solids at room temperature, but they are not the same. Coconut butter is the pureed meat of mature coconuts and is often thick and white. It has the fiber from the meat in it as well as some oil. Coconut oil has no fiber; the oil has been separated from the meat of the coconut. Coconut oil is often translucent and is more often used for cooking because it can be used for medium to high temperatures.

- Dark, leafy greens like Swiss chard and kale have a main vein that runs down the center of the leaf. This should be removed. Use scissors or cut with a knife to remove the vein.

- Vanilla extract is a liquid extract from the vanilla bean, whereas vanilla powder is the ground-up dried bean.

- When using lemon juice, use the juice of a lemon, not store-bought lemon juice. One lemon usually produces at least two tablespoons of juice.

Equipment and Tools Needed for Making Smoothies

Colander
Cutting board
Grater/Microplane/zester (only one is needed)
High-speed blender
Knife
Measuring cups
Measuring spoons
Vegetable peeler

MATCHA ENERGIZER

Matcha[1] tea provides a great boost of energy in this fiber- and protein-packed smoothie! Rich in antioxidants, it will keep you going all morning.

MAKES 2 TO 3 CUPS

½ teaspoon matcha tea powder

2 cups filtered water, divided

1 tablespoon vanilla extract

1 tablespoon coconut oil

1 cup almond milk

1 large handful spinach

2 tablespoons cashew butter

1 cup frozen raspberries

3–4 tablespoons hypoallergenic protein powder*

1 tablespoon unsweetened shredded coconut (optional)

1 tablespoon ground flaxseed (optional)

Such as the Gut C.A.R.E. CLEANSE SHAKE protein powder.

1. Combine the matcha tea powder and 1 tablespoon of the filtered water in a small ceramic bowl or mug and mix into a paste.

2. Heat 1 cup of the filtered water on the stovetop until fine bubbles form; do not boil. Add the heated water to the matcha paste and stir well to make tea. Set the tea aside and allow it to cool to room temperature.

3. In a blenderjar, combine the remaining filtered water and the rest of the ingredients in the order they are listed, including the coconut and flaxseed, if using. Add the cooled tea last.

4. Blend well on high for 20 to 30 seconds (until smooth).

5. Add a couple of ice cubes to the blender if you prefer to make your smoothie colder.

SWISS CHARD AND STRAWBERRY

Supergreen Swiss chard (the up-and-coming kale) makes this strawberry smoothie rich in nutrients and full of green fiber!

MAKES 2 TO 3 CUPS

1 heaping cup Swiss chard, main veins removed, chopped

2 large basil leaves

1¼ cups filtered water

1 tablespoon vanilla extract

1 tablespoon ground flaxseed

1 cup frozen strawberries

⅛ teaspoon lemon zest*

1 tablespoon coconut butter

3–4 tablespoons hypoallergenic protein powder

For lemon zest, use the small side of your grater, a lemon zester, or a micro-grater to shave the rind.

Add all the ingredients to a blender in the order they are listed. Blend well on high for 20 to 30 seconds.

RASPBERRY RECHARGE

Recharge with this slow-digesting raspberry-cashew-chia blend of healthy goodness . . . with superfood kale to boot!

MAKES 2 TO 3 CUPS

1 cup filtered water

1 vanilla rooibos tea bag*

½ cup kale (4 to 5 large leaves), roughly chopped

1 cup frozen raspberries

2 tablespoons cashew butter

1 cup almond milk

1 tablespoon ground chia seeds

1 tablespoon fresh lemon juice (about ½ lemon)

3–4 tablespoons hypoallergenic protein powder

Stevia extract, to taste (optional)

> *Any vanilla-flavored or fruity tea will work in place of vanilla rooibos if it is not available.*

1. Heat the filtered water on the stovetop, then remove from the heat, add the vanilla rooibos tea bag, and steep for at least 7 minutes. Set aside to cool.

2. Discard the tea bag, add the tea and the remaining ingredients, including the stevia, if using, to the blender in the order listed, and blend on high for 20 to 30 seconds.

3. Add a few ice cubes if you prefer a cooler smoothie.

Tips: The tea can be prepared the night before and placed in the refrigerator overnight so it is cool and ready to blend when you wake up. If you prepare it beforehand, make a big batch and use it whenever you are ready or want a refreshing iced tea. (Store in a glass bottle in the refrigerator for 3 to 5 days.) If you don't have time for the tea to cool, you can still use it when it is warm; just add some more ice to the smoothie at the end to cool down the temperature.

GO GREEN

A richly green, hydrating smoothie full of healthy fats and fiber. This fruit-free smoothie is a great go-to for overall health benefits!

MAKES 2 TO 3 CUPS

½ English cucumber*

1½ cups filtered water

1 teaspoon vanilla extract

⅛ teaspoon ground cinnamon

3 tablespoons fresh lemon juice (from 1 lemon)

10 walnut halves

1 tablespoon almond butter

1 teaspoon spirulina (available at any health-food store)

1 large handful baby spinach

¼ teaspoon sea salt

3–4 tablespoons hypoallergenic protein powder

1 tablespoon ground chia seeds (optional but recommended)

An English cucumber is longer and sometimes a bit thinner than a regular cucumber, and it has very tiny seeds. The English cucumber has a skin that is also very thin and does not need to be removed prior to eating. It can be found in the produce section of your local grocer, usually sold in plastic wrap. If you are using an English cucumber, simply cut in half, keeping the peel on, and trim off about ½ inch from the end. If you are not able to find an English cucumber, use any cucumber, but use a vegetable peeler to peel the skin off, cut the cucumber in half lengthwise, and use a spoon to scrape out and discard the seeds.

1. Add all the ingredients to a blender in the order listed. Blend until smooth.

2. Add a few ice cubes if you prefer a cooler smoothie.

SPICY AVOCADO

This smoothie is a spicy, stimulating treat that will keep you full for hours. Raw cacao and immunity-enhancing ginger make this smoothie antioxidant rich with a dose of healthy fat from the avocado.

MAKES 2 TO 3 CUPS

½ avocado, peeled and pit removed

1 cup almond milk

½ teaspoon ground cinnamon

2 teaspoons raw cacao powder

One 2-inch piece ginger, peeled and finely grated (about 1 tablespoon)

1 tablespoon coconut butter*

1 cup filtered water

1 tablespoon almond, sunflower, or cashew butter

½ cup kale (4 to 5 large leaves), main veins removed and roughly chopped

3–4 tablespoons hypoallergenic protein powder

Stevia extract, to taste (optional)

> *Coconut butter is found in most health-food stores. You can use it as is, no heating required.*

Add all the ingredients to a blender in the order listed and blend until smooth.

Tip: Peel ginger with a small paring knife, a vegetable peeler, or a teaspoon and grate with the small side of a grater or a Microplane.

BLUE GINGER

Mineral and phytonutrient rich, this smoothie features chlorella (a protein-filled, antioxidant-rich green algae), blueberries, and Brazil nuts. Great for your hair and skin!

MAKES 2 TO 3 CUPS

1 cup frozen blueberries
¼ cup whole Brazil nuts
1½ cups filtered water
2 teaspoons chlorella (available in powder form at health-food stores)
1 large handful spinach
One 2-inch piece ginger, peeled and finely grated (about 1 tablespoon)
1 tablespoon coconut oil
3–4 tablespoons hypoallergenic protein powder
¼ cup almond milk (optional; to help thin smoothie to desired consistency)

Add the ingredients to a blender in the order listed. Blend until smooth.

Tip: If you are not a fan of the strong bite of ginger, start with 1 teaspoon and add more as you desire. I love ginger and can never get enough.

CHOCOLATE-COVERED ALMOND

This protein-rich, healthy-fat-filled, chocolaty smoothie is a blood sugar–stabilizing treat!

MAKES 2 TO 3 CUPS

2 cups almond milk or coconut-almond milk

2 teaspoons raw cacao powder

2 tablespoons almond butter

1 teaspoon vanilla extract

1 teaspoon ground chia seeds

¼ teaspoon ground nutmeg

3–4 tablespoons hypoallergenic protein powder

¼ cup hemp hearts*

> *Hemp hearts are the shelled seeds of the hemp plant. They are an amazing superfood, rich in omega-3 fatty acids, protein, vitamins, and enzymes. You can find them at Whole Foods and many health-food stores.

1. Add all the ingredients to a blender in the order given. Blend until smooth.

2. Add a few ice cubes if you prefer a cooler smoothie.

HOMEMADE ALMOND MILK

A great alternative to cow's milk! Silky, fresh almond milk is best when made from scratch at home.

MAKES ABOUT 4 CUPS

1 cup raw, unsalted almonds
3 cups filtered water, plus filtered water for soaking the almonds
1 teaspoon vanilla powder, or 1 tablespoon vanilla extract
Pinch of sea salt

1. Soak the almonds overnight in filtered water.

2. Drain and rinse the almonds well and place in a blender.

3. Add the vanilla, sea salt, and 3 cups filtered water to the blender and blend on high for 20 to 30 seconds.

4. Pour the almond mixture from the blender through a fine-mesh strainer bag into a bowl.

5. Squeeze the bag over the bowl until all the almond milk is strained out.

6. Store for a maximum of 3 days in a glass bottle in the refrigerator, and shake before using, as the contents separate when they sit.

COCONUT-ALMOND MILK MADE FROM REAL COCONUT

My favorite! Coconut-almond milk made with fresh coconut meat and water adds an amazing natural sweetness while creating a wonderfully hydrating beverage.

MAKES ABOUT 4 CUPS

1 cup raw, unsalted almonds
3 cups filtered water, plus filtered water for soaking the almonds
1 fresh young coconut
1 teaspoon vanilla powder, or 1 tablespoon vanilla extract
Pinch of sea salt

1. Soak the almonds overnight in filtered water.

2. Drain and rinse the almonds well and place in a blender.

3. Open the coconut and add its water to the blender.

4. Use a spoon to peel out the coconut meat. Place it in a strainer and rinse well, getting all the woody tough parts off the meat. Add the coconut meat to the blender.

5. Add the vanilla, sea salt, and 3 cups filtered water to the blender and blend well.

6. Pour the almond-coconut mixture from the blender through a fine-mesh strainer bag into a bowl.

7. Squeeze the bag over the bowl until the almond-coconut milk is strained out.

8. Store in a glass bottle in the refrigerator for a maximum of 3 days, and shake before using, as the contents separate when they sit.

COCONUT-ALMOND MILK MADE FROM SHREDDED COCONUT

Homemade coconut-almond milk made with shredded coconut adds natural sweetness and creaminess to any beverage!

MAKES ABOUT 4 CUPS

1 cup raw, unsalted almonds
4 cups filtered water, plus filtered water for soaking the almonds
1 cup unsweetened shredded coconut (sulphate-free)
1 teaspoon vanilla powder or 3 teaspoons vanilla extract
Pinch of sea salt

1. Soak the almonds overnight in filtered water.

2. Heat 2 cups to just before boiling of the filtered water and add to a blender along with the shredded coconut. Allow to sit and soak for 30 minutes.

3. Drain and rinse the almonds well and place in the blender.

4. Add the vanilla, sea salt, and remaining 2 cups filtered water to the blender and blend well.

5. Pour the almond-coconut mixture from the blender through a fine-mesh strainer bag into a bowl.

6. Squeeze the bag over the bowl until the almond-coconut milk is strained out.

7. Store in a glass bottle in the refrigerator for a maximum of 3 days, and shake before using, as the contents separate when they sit.

COCONUT WATER KEFIR

A healthy prebiotic- and probiotic-rich carbonated beverage great for helping to balance your gut ecosystem.

MAKES 4 CUPS

3 tablespoons water kefir grains*

4 cups pasteurized coconut water

1 cup fresh strawberries or blueberries (optional)

½ cup fresh lemon juice (optional)

> *Water kefir grains can be found in natural-food stores or online at Amazon. With proper care, the culture can be used indefinitely to create probiotic-rich kefir. Your grains will not grow as quickly in coconut water as they will in a nice bath of nutrient-rich sugar. Refresh and reactivate the kefir grains in sugar water (¼ cup sugar in 4 cups water) for 24 to 48 hours between batches of Coconut Water Kefir. The sugar water will keep the grains healthy for the long term.

1. Place the water kefir grains and the coconut water in a jar. Cover the jar loosely with a lid or cheesecloth and allow the kefir grains to culture the coconut water for ideally 24 to 36 (and no longer than 48) hours at room temperature.

2. Once the culturing is complete (the mixture will have thickened), remove the kefir grains with a slotted spoon and store in a separate glass container filled with filtered water and a teaspoon of sugar to keep the kefir grains alive and active.

3. You may drink the Coconut Water Kefir by itself, but for an added twist, puree the cultured coconut water with the berries and lemon juice in a blender to your desired consistency. The Coconut Water Kefir will last 1 to 3 weeks in the fridge; when blended with the berries and lemon juice, it will last for 2 to 3 days in the fridge. Serve cold.

HOMEMADE VEGETABLE BROTH

A great staple to have on hand! Vegetable broth is used as a base in so many recipes, from soups to casseroles—even in stir-fries so you don't have to add as much oil.

MAKES 4 CUPS

4 carrots, roughly chopped

4 stalks celery, roughly chopped

½ medium zucchini, roughly chopped

½ medium parsnip, roughly chopped

4 green onions (green parts only), roughly chopped

5 bay leaves

1 tablespoon sea salt

1 teaspoon black pepper

½ cup fresh parsley

A few sprigs of fresh thyme

6 cups filtered water

1. Place all the vegetables, herbs, and seasonings in a large stockpot. Cover with the water. Bring to a boil, reduce the heat, and simmer for about 1 hour.

2. Pour the broth through a strainer to remove the solids. Store the broth in a mason jar in the refrigerator for a maximum of 3–4 days, or freeze for up to 3 months.

Tip: This keeps well in the freezer, too. I like to freeze the broth in ice cube trays and save it for recipes that require a small amount of vegetable broth.

IMMUNE-BOOSTING VEGETABLE SOUP

A delicious, low-calorie option to add to any meal or to have as a snack. Using a combination of multicolored veggies, medicinal mushrooms, and warming spices provides protective nutrients and phytochemicals to support a healthy immune response.

SERVES 8

2 cups Homemade Vegetable Broth (page 260)
4 cups Swiss chard, chopped
½ cup shiitake mushrooms
2 carrots, sliced
2 stalks celery, sliced
4 green onions, chopped
2 organic sweet potatoes, chopped
One 2-inch piece fresh ginger, peeled and thinly sliced
2 teaspoons sea salt
¼ teaspoon black pepper
1 teaspoon ground turmeric
2 cups filtered water

1. Combine all the ingredients in a large pot and cook over low heat for about 1½ hours, until all the veggies are soft.

2. Let the soup cool slightly, then blend with an immersion blender until creamy.

Tip: Any favorite combination of vegetables can be used in this recipe for a delicious, satisfying, and healthful soup. I sometimes throw in any leftover veggies I have in the refrigerator. You can substitute reishi or maitake mushrooms for the shiitakes; they are all rich in immune-boosting 1,3 beta-glucans.

GRASS-FED BEEF-BONE BROTH

Nutrition dense and loaded with flavor. Drink 8 ounces of this warm broth daily for its gut-healing properties. You can have it as part of your lunch or dinner.

MAKES 10 TO 15 SERVINGS

About 4 pounds grass-fed beef marrow bones
3 to 4 pounds grass-fed beef rib or neck bones with meat (optional)
½ cup fresh lemon juice or apple cider vinegar
1 to 2 teaspoons sea salt
½ teaspoon black pepper
Filtered water, as needed
3 stalks celery, roughly chopped
½ whole onion
1 bouquet garni (4 sprigs fresh thyme, 4 sprigs fresh rosemary, and 1 bunch
   parsley tied with unbleached string or a recycled tea bag string)

1. Combine the marrow bones and rib bones, if using, with the lemon juice, salt, and pepper in a large pot or slow cooker. Add filtered water to cover.

2. Cook for at least 4 hours on very low heat until any meat that was still on the bones has fallen off and the marrow has dissolved. You can cook the broth for up to 24 hours on low heat or in a slow cooker on low. You may need to add additional water; most important is that all the meat and marrow has fallen off the bones.

3. Add the celery, onion, and bouquet garni to the pot and cook for at least 1 to 2 hours more.

4. Pour the broth through a strainer to remove all the solid ingredients.

5. Store 5 cups of the broth in a glass container in the refrigerator for use during the week, and store the rest in a plastic-topped glass container in the freezer for future use.

Tip: Other veggies such as carrots, turnips, and squash can be added to give more flavor to the broth if desired. I usually make a week's worth of broth at a time so I have it ready whenever I want it.

PUMPKIN SOUP WITH COCONUT CREAM

A smooth and creamy soup. Delicious on a cool fall evening.

SERVES 4

FOR THE PUMPKIN SOUP

1 small whole organic pie pumpkin*

1 tablespoon organic ghee

1 teaspoon sea salt, divided

¼ teaspoon black pepper

1 tablespoon olive oil

1 shallot, minced

2 cups Homemade Vegetable Broth (page 260)

2 tablespoons maple syrup

½ cup unsweetened coconut milk

¼ teaspoon ground nutmeg

> *You can use one 15-ounce BPA-free can of organic pumpkin puree (such as the Farmer's Market brand) if you do not have fresh pumpkin.*

FOR THE COCONUT CREAM

¼ cup coconut milk

½ teaspoon ground cinnamon

1 teaspoon maple syrup

TO MAKE THE PUMPKIN SOUP

1. Preheat the oven to 300°F.

2. Cut the pumpkin in half and scrape out the seeds and pulp. Brush the pumpkin flesh with the ghee and sprinkle with ½ teaspoon of the salt and the pepper. Place the pumpkin halves, cut side facing down, on a baking sheet and roast for 45 minutes to 1 hour, or until tender.

3. Allow the pumpkin to cool slightly. Scoop out the flesh into a bowl and set aside.

4. Heat the olive oil in a large pot over medium heat. Add the shallot and cook for 5 minutes, until softened.

5. Add the vegetable broth, maple syrup, and pumpkin flesh to the pot and heat until simmering. Mash up any large pumpkin chunks, then transfer the mixture to a blender or food processor (or use an immersion blender) and puree until smooth. Return the mixture to the pot and add the coconut milk, nutmeg, and remaining ½ teaspoon salt. Continue to cook until heated through.

TO MAKE THE COCONUT CREAM

6. Whisk the coconut milk with the cinnamon and maple syrup.

TO SERVE

7. Pour the soup into serving bowls. Swirl in the coconut cream.

BUTTERNUT SQUASH BISQUE
WITH TOASTED WALNUTS

Roasting the vegetables brings out the intensity of their flavors in this hearty soup.

SERVES 8

1 large butternut squash, peeled, seeded, and chopped into ½-inch cubes*
2 cups organic whole baby carrots
1 medium sweet onion, diced
1 large sweet potato, peeled and cut into ½-inch pieces
1 tablespoon minced garlic
3 tablespoons walnut oil
Kosher salt, to taste
Black pepper, to taste
6 cups reduced-sodium, gluten-free, free-range chicken broth (homemade or
   store bought)
2 bay leaves
1½ cups unsweetened coconut milk
¼ cup chopped walnuts

> *Pumpkin or acorn squash also work well.*

1. Preheat the oven to 375°F.

2. In a medium bowl, toss all the vegetables with the walnut oil and salt and pepper to taste. Arrange on a baking sheet and roast for about 40 minutes, stirring occasionally, until the vegetables are soft and golden brown.

3. Place the roasted vegetables in a large pot and add the chicken broth. Add the bay leaves and bring to a boil. Lower the heat and simmer, covered, for approximately 30 minutes; the vegetables should be soft and falling apart.

4. Let the soup cool a little (about 15 minutes) so you don't burn yourself. Remove the bay leaves and puree the soup with an immersion blender. Place the pot back over medium heat.

5. Stir in the coconut milk until combined and check the seasonings. If the soup is too thick, add a little more chicken broth to obtain the desired consistency. Set aside.

6. Toast the walnuts in a skillet over low heat for about 3 minutes.

7. Serve the soup in individual bowls garnished with the toasted walnuts.

Tip: I also like to use unsweetened Homemade Almond Milk (page 256) in place of the coconut milk.

SUMMER FRESH CITRUS SALAD WITH SLICED ALMONDS

A light and refreshing salad, loaded with vitamin C and antioxidants, that is perfect as a side dish or as a meal.

SERVES 4

1 fennel bulb, thinly sliced

2 medium red or golden beets, washed and cut into ¼-inch pieces

¼ medium red onion, thinly sliced

¼ cup cilantro, chopped

1 head organic butter lettuce, washed, drained, and torn into bite-size pieces*

¼ cup walnut oil

Juice of 2 lemons

1 teaspoon salt

¼ teaspoon black pepper

2 pink seedless grapefruits, peeled and broken into segments

2 large seedless oranges, peeled and broken into segments

3 tablespoons sliced almonds**

Any variety of lettuce can be used. As an alternative, I love organic baby romaine.
**Walnuts and pistachios are also great in place of the almonds.*

1. Toss together the fennel, beets, onion, cilantro, and lettuce in a medium bowl.

2. Whisk together the oil, lemon juice, salt, and pepper until blended. Pour the dressing over the salad and toss.

3. Place the salad on a large serving platter.

4. Arrange the grapefruit and orange segments over the salad, top with the sliced almonds, and serve.

MEDITERRANEAN CHICKPEA SALAD

An excellent vegetarian appetizer or entrée. Chickpeas are terrific for providing water-soluble fiber—a gut-balancing prebiotic.

SERVES 6

2 cups organic, canned chickpeas (choose a BPA-free can like Eden Organic garbanzo beans)
1 pint organic cherry or grape tomatoes, halved
4 green onions, chopped
Juice of 1 lemon
¼ cup olive oil
1½ cups small pitted black olives
¼ cup chopped cilantro*
¼ teaspoon black pepper
½ teaspoon sea salt
Chopped parsley, for garnish

Any fresh herbs, such as basil, oregano, and parsley, may also be used.

1. Combine all the ingredients, except the parsley, in a medium bowl. Chill until ready to serve.

2. Garnish with the chopped parsley before serving.

Tip: Other chopped veggies may be added to the salad, such as carrots, cucumbers, and peppers.

AVOCADO AND ORGANIC
HEIRLOOM TOMATO SALAD

Summer-fresh heirloom tomatoes served with creamy avocado will refresh you. I love heirloom tomatoes, but if you have an arthritic condition, it's best to stay away from the nightshades, including tomatoes. Instead, just make this as an avocado salad, rich in anti-inflammatory omega-3s.

SERVES 4

FOR THE DRESSING
¼ cup cider vinegar
4 tablespoons walnut oil
1 teaspoon sea salt
¼ teaspoon black pepper
¼ teaspoon stevia extract

FOR THE SALAD
4 organic heirloom tomatoes, sliced into ¼-inch circles*
4 avocados, peeled, pitted, and chopped into large chunks*
1 small red onion, chopped

> *It is important to use fresh ripe tomatoes and avocados. Organic grape tomatoes can be sliced in half and tossed with the avocado and red onion if heirloom tomatoes are unavailable.*

1. Whisk all the dressing ingredients together in a small bowl until well combined. Taste and adjust the seasonings if desired. Set aside.

2. On a large platter, layer the tomatoes.

3. Arrange the diced avocado and onion over the tomatoes.

4. Drizzle the dressing over the salad and serve.

SHREDDED CARROT SALAD WITH TOASTED ALMONDS AND BERRIES

Here's a crispy, sweet salad that tastes like a treat while also being healthy for your gut and low in sugar.

SERVES 4

FOR THE DRESSING
¼ cup olive oil
3 tablespoons fresh lemon juice
1½ teaspoons brown mustard
1 teaspoon salt
¼ teaspoon stevia extract
Dash of ground cinnamon

FOR THE SALAD
One 10-ounce bag shredded carrots
½ cup blueberries*
¼ cup unsalted slivered almonds*

Other berries or nuts work nicely in this recipe as well.

1. Whisk together the ingredients for the dressing in a small bowl until well combined. Set aside.

2. Combine the carrots and blueberries in a medium bowl.

3. Toast the almonds for 3 to 4 minutes in a small skillet, taking care not to burn.

4. Toss the carrots and blueberries with the dressing, top with the almonds, and serve.

Tip: This salad will keep well for 1 to 2 days in the refrigerator.

MIXED GREENS WITH SLICED STRAWBERRIES

This is a light salad that is perfect with almost any meal. Strawberries help reduce bloating from water retention.

SERVES 4

FOR THE DRESSING
3 tablespoons walnut oil
1 tablespoon cider vinegar
2 tablespoons fresh-squeezed orange juice
1 teaspoon sea salt
⅛ teaspoon black pepper

FOR THE SALAD
1 large head organic butter lettuce, torn into 2-inch pieces
4 cups mixed organic mesclun greens
2 cups strawberries, sliced*

> *Blackberries, blueberries, and raspberries are also excellent in place of the strawberries. The key to this recipe is using sweet, delicious berries in season.

1. Whisk all the ingredients for the dressing together in a small bowl until well combined. Set aside.

2. Combine the lettuce and greens in a large bowl.

3. Toss the lettuce and greens with the dressing. Add the strawberries, toss, and serve.

CHICKEN AND PISTACHIO LETTUCE WRAPS

This is a super-flavorful way to have a breadless wrap, and the pistachios add a delightful savory crunch.

SERVES 4

FOR THE DRESSING

¼ cup olive oil

3 tablespoons cider vinegar

2 teaspoons dry mustard

1 teaspoon ground ginger

¼ teaspoon sea salt

¼ teaspoon black pepper

2 tablespoons minced fresh parsley

1 teaspoon grated lime zest

FOR THE CHICKEN AND PISTACHIO WRAPS

One 8-ounce free-range boneless, skinless chicken breast

¼ teaspoon sea salt

Three ¼-inch-thick slices fresh ginger, plus ¼ teaspoon grated fresh ginger

1 cup chopped English cucumber*

2 green onions (green parts only), thinly sliced

3 tablespoons fresh lime juice

2 tablespoons minced fresh parsley

12 leaves Bibb lettuce

¼ cup pistachios, finely chopped

English cucumbers are sweeter with smaller seeds and thinner skins than regular cucumbers. They are usually wrapped in plastic and unwaxed. You can use regular cucumber in this recipe; just peel the skin and remove the seeds.

1. Place all the dressing ingredients in a jar. Screw on the lid tightly and shake the dressing until well blended.

2. Place the chicken, salt, and sliced ginger in a saucepan. Cover with water and bring the liquid to a boil. Immediately reduce the heat to a bare simmer so that only an occasional bubble breaks the surface. At this point, partly cover the pot, cook for about 10 minutes, and then turn off the heat and cover the pot with a tight-fitting lid. Leave the chicken to finish cooking in the hot water for another 15 to 20 minutes, depending on the size of the chicken breast, until cooked through. Drain the liquid and remove the ginger pieces. Shred the chicken when cool enough to handle and set aside.

3. Place the cucumber, green onions, grated ginger, lime juice, and parsley in a large bowl. Add the chicken and mix together.

4. Divide the chicken mixture evenly among the 12 lettuce leaves. Sprinkle with the pistachios.

5. Drizzle the dressing on top of the lettuce wraps.

VEGGIE SLAW WITH CITRUS VINAIGRETTE

The perfect side to any meat dish. This is a great way to add more low-calorie veggies to your meal.

SERVES 4

FOR THE DRESSING

¼ cup fresh-squeezed orange juice

2 tablespoons cider vinegar

2 tablespoons walnut oil

1 teaspoon honey

2 teaspoons caraway seeds

½ teaspoon salt

¼ teaspoon black pepper

FOR THE SALAD

2 medium zucchini*

1 organic green apple, peeled, cored, and thinly sliced

> *Sweet peppers, shredded carrots, and cabbage also work well in addition to the zucchini.*

1. In a small bowl, whisk all the dressing ingredients together until well combined. Taste and adjust the seasonings if needed. Set aside.

2. Slice the zucchini in half lengthwise and scoop out the seeds with a spoon.

3. Using a vegetable peeler, peel the zucchini into long strips. Combine the zucchini strips and apple slices in a large bowl.

4. Toss the zucchini and apple with the dressing and mix together thoroughly.

5. Cover the bowl with a plate and refrigerate for at least 30 minutes. Toss again and enjoy!

Tip: Add extra seasonings, if desired, and toss in the nuts of your choice for a crunchy bonus.

WATERCRESS AND JICAMA SALAD

A peppery citrus salad that bursts with crunchy flavor.

SERVES 4

FOR THE DRESSING
¼ cup olive oil
1 tablespoon cider vinegar
2 tablespoons fresh orange juice
1 tablespoon fresh lime juice
¼ teaspoon sea salt
⅛ teaspoon black pepper

FOR THE SALAD
1 bunch watercress, trimmed and coarsely chopped
1¼ cups jicama, peeled and julienned*
½ cup fresh parsley, finely chopped
1 tablespoon chopped fresh mint leaves

Jicama is a root vegetable that is mild in flavor. It can be found in the produce section of your supermarket or in Latin American markets.

1. Combine all the dressing ingredients in a jar. Cover tightly with a lid and shake until the dressing is well blended. Set aside.

2. Combine the watercress, jicama, and parsley in a small salad bowl.

3. Pour the dressing over the salad, sprinkle with the mint leaves, and serve.

QUINOA SALAD WITH APPLES AND WALNUTS

Crunchy and sweet and fabulous! Quinoa, actually an edible seed, is a quick-and-easy-to-prepare gluten-free alternative that contains more protein than other grains.

SERVES 4

FOR THE DRESSING

¼ cup organic honey

2 tablespoons cider vinegar

¼ teaspoon dry mustard

¼ teaspoon sea salt

¼ cup flaxseed oil

FOR THE SALAD

2 cups filtered water

¼ cup fresh lemon juice

1 cup dry organic quinoa, rinsed

1 large green organic apple, chopped into bite-size pieces

2 green onions (green part only), thinly sliced

¼ cup chopped celery

¼ cup walnuts, toasted and chopped

2 cups salad greens

1. Combine all the dressing ingredients in a jar with a lid. Cover and shake until the ingredients are fully mixed. Set aside.

2. Bring the water and the lemon juice to a boil in a medium saucepan. Add the quinoa and reduce the heat to a simmer. Cover and simmer for 15 to 20 minutes until the water has been absorbed and the quinoa is tender. Remove from the heat and let stand, covered, for 5 minutes. Fluff with a fork and place in the refrigerator to chill for 5 to 10 minutes.

3. Combine the apple, green onions, celery, walnuts, and chilled quinoa in a large salad bowl and mix thoroughly.

4. Place the salad greens in a large serving bowl.

5. Stir the dressing into the quinoa mixture and serve over the salad greens.

Tip: Add grilled chicken or shrimp to make this a meal.

DR. PEDRE'S SCALLION VINAIGRETTE

I love this vinaigrette on top of almost everything. Terrific on salads, meats, and roasted veggies.

MAKES 1 CUP

1 to 2 small scallions (green onions), cut into ⅛-inch slices
⅔ cup cold-pressed extra-virgin olive oil
⅓ cup cider vinegar
2 teaspoons fresh lemon juice (about ½ lemon)
½ teaspoon Himalayan sea salt, to taste
¼ teaspoon freshly ground black pepper, to taste
Dried basil or herbes de Provence, to taste (optional)

1. Place the scallions in a large measuring cup or a mason jar.

2. Using a wooden spoon or a pestle, crush the scallions to release their juices and flavor.

3. Add the remaining ingredients and mix vigorously with a spoon or whisk, or place the lid on the mason jar, if using, and shake vigorously to distribute the ingredients evenly.

4. Serve on salads or use as a dressing on meat dishes.

Tips: Experiment with flavor by adding a little extra vinegar and/or lemon juice for a more refreshingly acidic marinade for meats, or less vinegar and/or lemon juice for a subtler dressing. The amount of dressing made can also be reduced or increased, as long as the proportions for each ingredient are maintained. For other flavor variations, add a favorite dried herb or mixture of herbs to taste.

FLAX SUPER-SEED CRACKERS

Loaded with fiber, trace minerals, and healthy fats, these crackers are great for serving on the side with salads and soups or as a quick snack between meals.

MAKES 20 CRACKERS (10 SERVINGS)

2 cups ground flaxseed*
1 cup filtered water, divided
2 tablespoons hulled pumpkin seeds
2 tablespoons hulled sunflower seeds
2 tablespoons hulled sesame seeds
½ teaspoon salt
½ teaspoon black pepper
Dash of cayenne pepper (optional)

You can use ground chia or sesame seeds in place of the flaxseed.

1. Preheat the oven to 400°F. Line a baking sheet with parchment paper.

2. In a large bowl, combine the flaxseed and ½ cup of the water. Mix together until a dough begins to form.

3. Gradually add up to ½ cup additional water to moisten the dough and make it more workable; make sure the dough does not become too wet.

4. Mix in the pumpkin, sunflower, and sesame seeds until they are evenly distributed.

5. Spread out the dough on the baking sheet so it is approximately ⅛ to ¼ inch thick. Sprinkle the dough evenly with the salt and pepper; add cayenne, if desired, for an extra kick of spice.

6. Cut the dough into 20 squares and bake for 20 to 30 minutes or until the crackers are crisp and the edges are browned.

7. Store in an airtight container.

NUT AND SEED BARS

A power-packed, fiber-rich snack.

MAKES 8 SNACK BARS

½ cup raw almonds*
½ cup walnuts*
2 tablespoons chia seeds*
2 tablespoons hemp seeds*
2 tablespoons ground flaxseed*
1 tablespoon raw hulled pumpkin seeds*
1 tablespoon hulled sunflower seeds*
1 tablespoon coconut oil
1 tablespoon ground cinnamon
1 teaspoon vanilla extract
¾ cup almond butter

> *Use any combination of nuts (such as chopped brazil nuts) and seeds (such as sesame) in these bars.*

1. Place all the ingredients, except the almond butter, in a high-powered blender or a food processor. Mix until combined and finely chopped.

2. Add the almond butter and process until the mixture forms a ball.

3. Line an 8-by-8-inch pan with parchment paper. Press the mixture into the pan and refrigerate for about 1 hour.

4. Slice and serve. Store, covered, in the refrigerator.

Tip: You can also add 1 cup dairy-free, soy-free, and gluten-free chocolate chips (such as Enjoy Life Foods Dark Chocolate Morsels) as an option.

CRISPY KALE CHIPS

Crispy, flavorful, and loaded with vitamin C, iron, and fiber.

SERVES 4

4 to 6 cups kale (about 1 nice-sized bunch of kale or 1 bag of fresh kale leaves)
1½ tablespoons olive oil
1 teaspoon garlic powder
Sea salt, to taste
Cayenne pepper or chipotle chili powder, to taste (optional)

1. Preheat the oven to 300°F. Line a baking sheet with aluminum foil.

2. If you purchased a bunch of kale rather than bagged kale, remove the leaves from the bunch and discard the stems.

3. Wash the kale in a colander and squeeze out the excess water with a paper towel.

4. Place the kale in a bowl. Add the olive oil and mix by hand to coat each kale leaf.

5. Lay out the kale leaves on the baking sheet so that they are flat and not overlapping.

6. Sprinkle on the garlic powder, sea salt, and other seasonings, if using, and bake for 10 minutes or until the leaves are crispy. Taste and add additional seasonings as desired.

Tip: Keep a close eye on your kale chips as they are baking because they can burn fairly quickly!

MAHI-MAHI WITH SHALLOTS, LIME, AND VEGGIES IN PARCHMENT

A versatile, easy-to-prepare meal with little to no cleanup!

SERVES 2

Two 6-ounce wild mahi-mahi fillets (about 1 inch thick)*

½ teaspoon sea salt

¼ teaspoon black pepper

1 tablespoon coconut oil

1 teaspoon grated lime zest

1 tablespoon fresh lime juice

1 tablespoon minced fresh parsley**

1 tablespoon minced fresh thyme**

1 shallot, minced**

½ cup julienned carrots**

½ cup julienned snow peas**

½ cup julienned zucchini**

4 thin slices lime

> *Use any firm-fleshed wild white fish fillet such as halibut, cod, or haddock.
> **You may also try different combinations of herbs and vegetables.

1. Preheat the oven to 400°F.

2. Cut two 15-by-24-inch pieces of parchment paper. Fold in half crosswise. Draw half a large heart on each piece, with the fold of the paper along the center of the heart. Using scissors, cut out two heart-shaped pieces of parchment.

3. Sprinkle the fish with the salt and pepper. Place one fillet near the fold of each parchment heart.

4. Combine the coconut oil, lime zest, lime juice, parsley, and thyme in a bowl; stir until blended.

5. Top each fillet with half of the coconut oil mixture. Evenly divide the shallot, carrots, snow peas, and zucchini between the two fillets, and top with 2 lime slices apiece.

6. Starting at the top of the heart, fold one half of the heart over the other, fully covering the fish. Seal the edges with narrow folds. Twist the end tip to secure tightly.

7. Place the parchment packets on a baking sheet. Bake for 15 minutes. Transfer to serving plates, cut open the parchment paper, and serve immediately.

STIR-FRIED VEGGIES AND SHRIMP OVER RICE NOODLES

A quick-and-easy weekday meal. With gut-soothing ghee, this rich combination of shrimp, veggies, and noodles really satisfies your palate.

SERVES 4

8 ounces dry rice noodles

1 pound large wild raw shrimp, peeled and deveined

1¼ teaspoons sea salt, divided

¼ teaspoon black pepper

2 tablespoons ghee, divided*

1 cup mushrooms, sliced**

1 cup shredded carrots**

1 cup pea pods**

2 small green onions, thinly sliced**

1 cup Homemade Vegetable Broth (page 260)

1 tablespoon cider vinegar

2 teaspoons molasses

½ teaspoon ground ginger

1 tablespoon sesame oil

¼ cup fresh basil, chopped

1 tablespoon toasted sesame seeds

> *If you don't have ghee, avocado or coconut oil is a great substitute.
> **Use any combination of vegetables in this dish.

1. Bring a pot of water to a boil. Add the rice noodles, remove from the heat, and let sit for 5 minutes until tender. Drain and rinse the noodles in cold water, and set aside.

2. Sprinkle the shrimp with ½ teaspoon of the sea salt and ¼ teaspoon of the pepper.

3. Heat 1 tablespoon of the ghee in a large skillet over medium-high heat. Sauté the shrimp in the skillet until firm and pink, 5 to 10 minutes. Transfer the shrimp to a platter.

4. Reduce the heat to medium and add the remaining 1 tablespoon ghee. Add the mushrooms, carrots, pea pods, and green onions. Sauté until tender, 2 to 3 minutes.

5. In a small bowl, whisk together the vegetable broth, vinegar, molasses, remaining ¾ teaspoon sea salt, ginger, and sesame oil. Add the sauce to the vegetables in the skillet. Stir in the rice noodles and shrimp and continue to cook until heated through.

6. Sprinkle with the basil and sesame seeds and serve hot or cold.

ROASTED WILD SALMON WITH DILL SAUCE

A rich, satisfying meal loaded with omega-3 fatty acids and calcium.

SERVES 4

FOR THE SALMON
One 1-pound wild salmon fillet
¼ teaspoon sea salt
⅛ teaspoon black pepper

FOR THE DILL SAUCE
2 tablespoons organic ghee*
2 tablespoons unsweetened coconut milk
1 tablespoon ground cashews
¼ cup fresh dill, chopped
2 tablespoons chopped fresh chives
2 cloves garlic, chopped
1 teaspoon Dijon mustard
½ teaspoon stevia extract (optional)
½ teaspoon sea salt
¼ teaspoon black pepper

If you don't have ghee, refined coconut oil is a great substitute.

TO MAKE THE SALMON
1. Preheat the oven to 450°F.

2. Wash and dry the salmon with paper towels. Run your hands over the salmon and feel for any bones; if found, pull out with your fingertips or with a pair of clean, needle-nose pliers.

3. Place the salmon skin side down in a roasting pan, sprinkle with the salt and pepper, and bake for 15 to 22 minutes, until the salmon flakes easily with a fork.

TO MAKE THE DILL SAUCE

4. In a medium saucepan over low heat, heat the ghee. Add the coconut milk and cashews and heat for 2 to 3 minutes, until the mixture starts to thicken a little. With a spoon, stir in the dill, chives, garlic, and mustard and cook for about 3 minutes more. Add the stevia (if desired), salt, and pepper.

5. Serve the sauce over the baked salmon.

Tips: Salmon also cooks well when wrapped in an aluminum foil packet. You can add a little lemon juice to the sauce to add some extra flavor.

ROASTED CHICKEN

A great low-calorie meal, a roasted chicken is easy to prepare and makes a rich and satisfying meal with plenty of leftovers (if cooking for yourself).

SERVES 6

One 5- to 6-pound whole chicken
2 teaspoons sea salt
½ teaspoon black pepper
1 teaspoon ground turmeric
½ teaspoon paprika
2 tablespoons chopped fresh thyme
¼ cup parsley sprigs
Juice of 1 lemon
2 tablespoons organic ghee
2 teaspoons garlic powder
1 teaspoon onion powder
1 medium Spanish onion, cut into 1-inch pieces
1 cup whole baby carrots
1 cup filtered water

1. Preheat the oven to 425°F.

2. Remove the bag of giblets from inside the chicken cavity and discard.[2] Drain any excess fluids.

3. Wash the outside of the chicken and trim off any excess fat.

4. Pat the entire chicken down with paper towels until dry. Tie the legs together with cooking string and tuck the wing tips under the body of the chicken.

5. Place the chicken in a roasting pan and sprinkle with the salt, pepper, turmeric, and paprika.

6. Place the thyme and parsley into the chicken cavity.

7. Drizzle the lemon juice and ghee over the chicken, and sprinkle with the garlic and onion powders.

8. Surround the chicken with the onion and carrots. Pour the water into the roasting pan.

9. Roast the chicken for about 1½ hours, basting frequently, until the leg feels like it would pull easily away from the chicken, or a meat thermometer inserted into the chicken thigh reads 165°F.

10. Serve with the carrots and onion.

Tips: This roasting method works well with any game bird. You can also use the cooking juices and simmer them down in a separate saucepan to make an excellent gravy.

CHICKEN PICCATA

This flavorful, lemony chicken is perfect for any occasion.

SERVES 4

1 pound free-range, antibiotic-free chicken tenderloins, cleaned*
⅓ cup brown rice flour
½ teaspoon salt
¼ teaspoon black pepper
¼ cup organic ghee**
2 shallots, chopped
3 tablespoons fresh lemon juice
2 tablespoons capers
¾ cup chicken broth
Lemon twists, to garnish (slice lemons into thin rounds, make a cut halfway
 through the round, and give it a twist)

Turkey or pork cutlets also work well in place of the chicken tenderloins.
***Olive oil can be substituted for the ghee.**

1. Place the chicken tenderloins in a single layer between two sheets of parchment paper and pound until about ¼ inch thick.

2. Mix together the rice flour, salt, and pepper in a shallow bowl.

3. Dip the chicken tenderloins into the flour mixture, coating each side evenly.

4. Heat the ghee in a large skillet on medium heat for 2 to 3 minutes.

5. Turn the heat to medium-high and add half the chicken pieces in a single layer; do not crowd. Cook for 4 to 5 minutes on each side, until the chicken is light brown; remove and set aside. Cook the remaining chicken pieces in the same manner; remove and set aside with the first batch.

6. Add the shallots to the pan and sauté for 2 minutes.

7. Add the lemon juice, capers, chicken broth, and chicken pieces to the same pan. Simmer for about 5 minutes until the sauce thickens.

8. Transfer the chicken piccata to a serving dish and garnish with the lemon twists. Serve.

Tip: This dish can be made 2 to 3 days ahead; it reheats beautifully.

STUFFED MEXICAN TURKEY BURGER

These Paleo-style burgers are bursting with flavor from the Cilantro Pesto.

MAKES 4 BURGERS

1 pound ground turkey

2 tablespoons unsweetened coconut milk

½ teaspoon sea salt

1 teaspoon ground cumin

1 teaspoon ground coriander

1 teaspoon dried cilantro

1 teaspoon dried oregano

Cilantro Pesto (recipe follows)

12 large butter lettuce leaves

1 avocado, sliced

1. Preheat the oven to 400°F. Line a rimmed baking sheet with parchment paper.

2. In a mixing bowl, combine the turkey, coconut milk, salt, cumin, coriander, cilantro, and oregano. Form into 8 patties.

3. Place 4 patties on the baking sheet. Put 1 tablespoon Cilantro Pesto in the center of each patty. Top with the remaining 4 patties, pressing the edges to seal.

4. Bake for 20 minutes. Remove the patties when done and place each burger on 3 large butter lettuce leaves. Top with the sliced avocado and drizzle with the remaining pesto.

Tip: These burgers can be cooked on the stovetop in a grill pan or on an outside barbecue grill.

CILANTRO PESTO

Cilantro brings in a tangy, delicious taste to any recipe and adds a terrific Latin flair.

MAKES ABOUT ⅔ CUP

1 cup lightly packed fresh cilantro
1 tablespoon unsalted, hulled pumpkin seeds
¼ teaspoon sea salt
¼ teaspoon black pepper
1 tablespoon fresh lemon juice
2 tablespoons olive oil

Place the cilantro, pumpkin seeds, salt, pepper, and lemon juice in a food processor. With the processor running, slowly add the olive oil. Process until smooth.

CHICKEN CURRY

This is an easy-to-prepare, fragrant, and flavorful dish!

SERVES 4

2 tablespoons coconut oil, divided

1 pound boneless, skinless chicken breast, cut into ¼-inch strips

½ teaspoon sea salt

3 green onions (green part only), thinly sliced

2 teaspoons ground turmeric

1 teaspoon ground cumin

1 teaspoon ground coriander

1 teaspoon dried cilantro

1 teaspoon ground ginger

½ teaspoon ground mustard

½ teaspoon ground cardamom

¼ teaspoon black pepper

¼ teaspoon ground cinnamon

¼ teaspoon ground cloves

¾ cup coconut milk

1. Heat 1 tablespoon of the coconut oil in a large skillet over medium-high heat.

2. Sprinkle the chicken with the salt and add to the skillet in a single layer. Cook, stirring occasionally, until lightly browned but still pink in spots, about 3 minutes. Transfer the partially cooked chicken to a clean bowl and set aside.

3. Add the remaining 1 tablespoon coconut oil to the pan. Add the sliced green onion. Blend together all the spices in a separate bowl, then add to the skillet. Cook until fragrant, about 1 minute.

4. Stir in the coconut milk. Reduce the heat to a simmer. Add the partially cooked chicken. Cover and simmer for about 15 minutes. Serve.

Tips: Stir in organic green peas for added color and flavor. Serve over brown basmati rice or Coconut Brown Rice (page 302).

GRASS-FED BEEF AND LAMB ENTRÉES

BEEF KABOBS

Quick and easy, this is the perfect barbecue meal.

SERVES 4

1 pound grass-fed sirloin steak, cut into 2-inch pieces
3 tablespoons olive oil
1 teaspoon sea salt
½ teaspoon black pepper
2 cloves garlic, chopped
½ teaspoon ground cumin
½ teaspoon ground turmeric
2 bell peppers, cut into 2-inch pieces
1 large sweet onion, cut into 2-inch pieces
8 medium mushrooms

1. Place all the ingredients in a large, sealable plastic bag, seal, and toss. Refrigerate overnight.

2. Separate the meat, bell peppers, onion, and mushrooms. Alternately thread the ingredients on stainless-steel skewers. Use equal amounts of all the ingredients to make four skewers.

3. Preheat your grill and then turn down the heat to a medium flame.

4. Grill the kabobs until the meat is cooked to the desired doneness.

Tip: If you want to use softer vegetables as well, like cherry tomatoes or zucchini, precook the peppers and onions separately on the grill for about 3 minutes before placing them and the tomatoes and zucchini on the skewers. If you don't precook the harder vegetables, they will be raw when you remove them from the grill, and the tomatoes and zucchini will be overcooked.

BISON BURGER

Bison is an alternative meat that is leaner than beef and has become quite popular in recent years. This simple, flavorful meat is all that is needed for a truly great meal.

SERVES 4

1 pound grass-fed lean ground bison*
1 teaspoon sea salt
¼ teaspoon black pepper
2 tablespoons chopped fresh chives

> *Venison also makes a great burger; just substitute ground venison in place of the ground bison.*

1. Mix all the ingredients together thoroughly.

2. Form the meat into 4 tightly packed balls.

3. Flatten each meatball into a firmly pressed patty.

4. Grill or broil the patties until the meat is cooked the way you like it.

5. Serve on a gluten-free brown rice bun or a lettuce wrap with avocado slices, or alongside roasted veggies, like carrots, squash, and red onions.

Tip: Bison is best if cooked medium-rare to medium. Because it is lower in fat than beef, it will tend to dry out if cooked beyond medium.

ROSEMARY LAMB

This holiday favorite is easy to make and so tasty.

SERVES 8

3 tablespoons olive oil

3 cloves garlic, sliced

2 tablespoons chopped fresh rosemary

1 teaspoon black pepper

1 teaspoon sea salt

1 teaspoon grated lemon zest

One 5-pound leg of lamb

1. Preheat the oven to 450°F.

2. Heat the olive oil and garlic in a small saucepan over low heat until the garlic is softened and the oil is fragrant, about 5 minutes. Remove from the heat. Pour the oil through a strainer into a small bowl to remove all the garlic. Stir the rosemary, pepper, salt, and lemon zest into the oil.

3. Place the lamb on a rack in a roasting pan. Rub the oil mixture evenly over the lamb.

4. Roast for 20 minutes, then reduce the oven temperature to 400°F and roast for 55 to 60 more minutes for medium-rare, or 75 to 80 minutes for medium. The internal temperature of the lamb should be at least 145°F when taken with a meat thermometer. Place the meat thermometer in the thickest part of the lamb when you are checking the temperature. Let the roast rest for 10 minutes before carving.

5. Serve with Roasted Sweet Potato Wedges with Toasted Pumpkin Seeds (page 300) and your favorite steamed vegetables or a side salad.

Tip: To enhance the flavor, marinate the lamb with the oil and seasoning mixture for several hours in the refrigerator before roasting.

SEARED STEAK WITH DIJON-HORSERADISH SAUCE

The creamy sauce in this recipe will work well with any cut of steak.

SERVES 2

Two 1¼- to 1½-inch-thick grass-fed New York strip steaks (about 8 ounces each)
1 teaspoon sea salt
½ teaspoon black pepper
1 teaspoon olive oil
½ cup full-fat coconut milk
1 tablespoon Dijon mustard
1 tablespoon prepared horseradish
1 tablespoon chopped fresh chives

1. Remove the steaks from the refrigerator and let them come to room temperature, about 30 minutes.

2. Season the steaks on both sides with the salt and pepper. Rub both sides with the olive oil.

3. Heat a medium heavy-bottomed ceramic-coated frying pan over high heat until very hot, but not smoking, about 3 minutes. Place the steaks in the pan and cook undisturbed until a dark crust forms on the bottom, 3 to 4 minutes.

4. Flip the steaks over and cook until medium-rare, 3 to 4 more minutes. The steaks should be firm around the edges but still give in the center. (If you prefer your steaks rare, cook about 1 minute less on each side. For medium or well-done, cook for 1 to 2 minutes more on each side.)

5. Transfer the steaks to a cutting board and let rest for at least 5 minutes before serving.

6. In a small bowl, whisk together the coconut milk, mustard, and horseradish until slightly thickened, 2 to 3 minutes. Stir in the chives. Serve over the steaks.

ROASTED SWEET POTATO WEDGES WITH TOASTED PUMPKIN SEEDS

The combination of the sweet, firm potatoes with the crunchy pumpkin seeds is so yummy. This is a great side to accompany the Rosemary Lamb (page 298) as well as the Bison Burgers (page 297). Sometimes I eat this dish as a snack right out of the fridge.

SERVES 4

3 tablespoons olive oil, plus extra to coat the casserole dish
4 medium organic sweet potatoes, scrubbed, peeled, and cut into 2-inch
 wedges*
¼ teaspoon ground cinnamon
¼ teaspoon ground coriander
1½ teaspoons sea salt
Dash of black pepper
¼ cup hulled pumpkin seeds

> *Slices of peeled butternut squash may be used in place of the sweet potatoes.*

1. Preheat the oven to 425°F. Coat a casserole dish with olive oil.

2. Place the sweet potato wedges in a medium bowl and toss with the cinnamon, coriander, salt, and pepper. Add the olive oil and toss again until all the pieces are evenly coated.

3. Place the sweet potatoes in the prepared casserole dish.

4. Roast for about 35 minutes, until the potatoes are crisp on the outside but pierce easily with a fork.

5. While the potatoes are roasting, toast the pumpkin seeds in a skillet over medium heat for 3 to 4 minutes, taking care not to burn them.

6. Remove the roasted sweet potatoes from the oven, toss with the toasted pumpkin seeds, and serve.

Tip: The easiest way to cut the sweet potatoes is to cut them in half, then cut each half into a half, then cut each quarter into thirds.

COCONUT BROWN RICE

Coconut gives a slight hint of the tropics to this classic staple. I love it with fish, poultry, or even just steamed vegetables. Yum!

SERVES 4

2 tablespoons coconut oil
1 cup organic brown basmati or long-grain organic brown rice*
2½ cups filtered water
1 teaspoon sea salt
½ cup unsweetened shredded coconut

> *This recipe also works well with quinoa or millet substituted for the brown rice.

1. Heat the coconut oil in a 2-quart saucepan.

2. Add the rice to the pan and heat until the rice starts to brown a little and is fragrant.

3. Add the water to the pan and bring to a boil.

4. Lower the heat to the lowest setting and cover the saucepan; let the rice cook for 20 to 25 minutes.

5. Check to see that all the water has been absorbed; if not, cook a little longer, until all the liquid has been absorbed. If the rice seems too dense, add a bit more water.

6. When all the water has been absorbed and the rice is soft and fluffy, sprinkle in the salt and fold in the coconut.

7. Cook for 3 to 4 minutes more on low heat, remove from the stove, and serve.

SPAGHETTI SQUASH WITH GARLIC-INFUSED OIL AND PINE NUTS

A satisfying alternative to a traditional pasta dish. Spaghetti squash is so low in calories, yet contains a filling and rich blend of fiber, antioxidants, and phytonutrients.

SERVES 4

One 2-pound spaghetti squash
3 tablespoons olive oil, divided
½ teaspoon sea salt
¼ teaspoon black pepper
2 cloves garlic, sliced
¼ cup pine nuts, toasted*
1 teaspoon grated lemon zest
2 tablespoons fresh lemon juice
¼ cup fresh parsley, finely chopped

> *If you have an allergy to pine nuts, you can substitute slivered almonds, sesame seeds, or chopped walnuts.*

1. Preheat the oven to 375°F.

2. Prick the squash all over with a small, sharp knife.

3. Place the squash on a rimmed baking sheet and roast until tender when pierced with a knife, about 1 hour and 20 minutes, flipping halfway through.

4. Remove the squash from the oven and let it cool for about 25 minutes.

5. Cut the squash in half lengthwise. Scrape out the seeds and brush each half with ½ tablespoon of the olive oil. Season with the salt and pepper.

6. Scrape the inside of the squash with a fork to remove strands; set the strands aside.

7. In a small saucepan, heat the remaining 2 tablespoons olive oil with the garlic over low heat until the garlic is softened, about 5 minutes.

8. Pour the oil through a strainer into a small bowl and remove all the garlic.

9. Add the pine nuts to the oil in the bowl, crushing them lightly with the back of a fork. Add the lemon zest, lemon juice, and parsley.

10. Toss the squash with the lemon mixture and serve.

Tip: Because spaghetti squash is difficult to cut through when uncooked and to avoid using a microwave, the squash in this recipe is roasted whole before cutting.

BUCKWHEAT PASTA AND VEGETABLES IN HOMEMADE VEGETABLE BROTH

These flavorful noodles can be enjoyed hot or cold with any combination of your favorite vegetables.

SERVES 4

1 tablespoon olive oil

1 cup sliced green onions (green parts only)

½ cup chopped fresh chives, plus 1 tablespoon, to serve

½ cup finely chopped carrots

½ cup finely chopped celery

2 cups Homemade Vegetable Broth (page 260)*

1 cup baby carrots

1 cup broccoli florets

½ cup sliced zucchini

½ cup sliced yellow squash

8 ounces buckwheat noodles, cooked according to package directions, rinsed under cold water, and drained

¾ teaspoon sea salt

½ teaspoon black pepper

1 tablespoon chopped fresh parsley

1 tablespoon chopped fresh thyme

2 tablespoons toasted sesame seeds, to serve

1 tablespoon toasted hemp seeds, to serve

> *To save time, use organic, gluten-free prepared vegetable broth in place of homemade.

1. Heat the olive oil in a large saucepan over medium-high heat. Add the green onions, ½ cup chives, carrots, and celery. Sauté until softened, about 5 minutes.

2. Stir in the vegetable broth, carrots, broccoli, zucchini, and yellow squash. Cover and simmer for 10 to 15 minutes or until the vegetables are tender.

3. Stir in the noodles, salt, pepper, parsley, and thyme. Continue to simmer until heated through, about 5 minutes.

4. Sprinkle with the sesame seeds, hemp seeds, and remaining 1 tablespoon chives. Serve.

HARVEST WILD RICE BOWL

A yummy one-bowl meal makes a satisfying winter dish. Terrific served with Crispy Kale Chips (page 282).

SERVES 4

1 to 2 tablespoons olive oil, plus extra to coat the baking pan

1 medium butternut squash (4 to 5 cups after roasting)

Olive oil cooking spray

1 organic green apple, chopped

1 to 2 teaspoons stevia extract

¼ cup diced onion (optional)

3 cups fresh spinach

2 cups cooked gluten-free wild rice blend of your choice*

3 tablespoons cider vinegar

Cooked quinoa or millet also works well in this recipe.

1. Preheat the oven to 400°F. Lightly coat a baking pan with olive oil.

2. Slice the butternut squash down the middle lengthwise and scoop out the seeds.

3. Bake the squash, cut side facing down, in the prepared baking pan for about 1 hour or until the flesh is soft.

4. Coat a skillet with olive oil cooking spray and add the apple. Cook for 4 to 5 minutes on medium heat, stirring to avoid sticking. Sprinkle the stevia on top of the apple and continue to cook until slightly browned and a bit softened, 2 to 3 minutes. Place the apple chunks in a bowl and set aside.

5. Remove the squash from the oven and let it cool for about 25 minutes. Scoop out the squash flesh from the skin with a large spoon and place in a bowl. Set aside. Discard the skin.

6. Heat the olive oil in a large skillet over medium heat and sauté the onion, if using, until translucent.

7. Add the spinach to the skillet and cook until the leaves have wilted.

8. Add the squash, cooked wild rice, and apple to the skillet and give the mixture a stir.

9. Turn the heat to low and stir in the vinegar, allowing the mixture to simmer for 2 to 3 minutes. Remove from the stove and serve.

Tip: To peel the squash's thick skin, start by cutting 1 inch from the top and bottom. Then, using a serrated peeler, peel away the thick skin until you reach the deeper orange flesh of the squash.

Time-Saving Tip: To speed up the prep time, purchase a peeled and chopped butternut squash at your local grocery store. Steam it in a 360 Cookware sauté pan over medium-high heat for approximately 10 minutes until tender when pierced with a knife. Use enough water to cover only the bottom of the pan.

ROASTED CAULIFLOWER WITH TOASTED WALNUT TOPPING

An easy side dish to complement any meal. Cauliflower is in the cruciferous family—our anticancer superfoods.

SERVES 4

1 small head cauliflower (about 2¼ pounds), trimmed into small florets

4 teaspoons organic ghee, at room temperature and divided

1 tablespoon finely chopped fresh rosemary

½ teaspoon sea salt

¼ teaspoon black pepper

¼ cup walnuts, finely chopped

2 tablespoons chopped fresh parsley

½ teaspoon grated lemon zest

1. Preheat the oven to 450°F.

2. Toss the cauliflower florets with 3 teaspoons of the ghee, the rosemary, salt, and pepper. Spread the cauliflower in a single layer on a rimmed baking sheet.

3. Roast the cauliflower until tender and lightly browned, 25 to 30 minutes, stirring once or twice. Remove and set aside.

4. Meanwhile, toast the walnuts in a small skillet over medium heat, stirring until toasted, 3 to 4 minutes. Remove from the heat and stir in the remaining 1 teaspoon ghee, parsley, and lemon zest.

5. Sprinkle the walnut mixture over the cauliflower and serve.

Tip: Try a different herb, such as thyme or dill, in place of the rosemary to vary the flavor.

VEGGIE-STUFFED SPRING ROLLS

These spring rolls make a great appetizer, snack, or party food.

SERVES 8

One 3.75-ounce package bean
  threads
½ cup chopped green onions
2 cups fresh spinach, chopped
1 cup shredded green cabbage
½ cucumber, peeled and finely
  chopped
½ cup shredded carrots

½ cup fresh parsley, chopped
1 tablespoon toasted sesame seeds
2 tablespoons fresh lime juice
1 teaspoon grated fresh ginger
1 teaspoon sesame oil
16 rice paper spring roll wrappers
  (usually found in an Asian market)
16 fresh basil leaves

1. Soak the bean threads in warm water for 4 to 5 minutes until softened. Drain.

2. In a large bowl, toss together the bean threads, green onions, spinach, cabbage, cucumber, carrots, parsley, and sesame seeds.

3. In a small bowl, whisk together the lime juice, ginger, and sesame oil. Add the dressing to the bean thread mixture and mix well.

4. Submerge the spring roll wrappers in hot water until pliable, about 15 seconds. Place 1 basil leaf and 2 tablespoons of the bean thread mixture on each wrapper. Fold in the sides and roll up tightly.

Tips: Bean threads are also known as glass noodles or cellophane noodles. They can be found in Asian markets or in the international section of your regular supermarket, along with spring roll wrappers. Be creative and add other vegetables or even meats to make this a great go-to lunch meal.

COCONUT MACAROONS

Chewy, creamy, and loaded with coconut flavor! Who could ask for more when you need a little decadence in your life?

MAKES 12 COOKIES

1 tablespoon coconut oil, to coat the baking pan

½ tablespoon ground flaxseed

1½ tablespoons warm filtered water

1⅓ cups unsweetened shredded coconut (sulphate-free)

⅓ cup organic honey

3 to 4 tablespoons almond meal

½ teaspoon salt

½ teaspoon pure almond extract

1. Preheat the oven to 325°F. Coat a baking sheet with the coconut oil.

2. Combine the flaxseed and water in a cup and let sit for about 5 minutes until the mixture thickens slightly.

3. Mix the flax mixture with all the remaining ingredients until well combined. If the mixture is too wet, add a little almond meal; if too dry, add a little water.

4. Using a 1-tablespoon cookie scoop, place 12 large round macaroons on the baking sheet.

5. Bake for 10 to 12 minutes, until golden, taking care not to burn the bottoms of the cookies.

6. Remove the macaroons from the baking sheet with a spatula and place on aluminum foil to cool for 15 minutes. Store in an airtight container once cooled.

Tip: You can make a thumbprint in the center of each macaroon before baking and place a whole raw almond in the middle.

ALMOND-HEMP CHOCOLATE TRUFFLES

Delicious omega-3-rich chocolate bites to satisfy any sweet tooth.

MAKES 12 TRUFFLES

½ cup almond butter
6 tablespoons coconut oil, refrigerated until solid
½ cup hemp seeds
½ cup almond flour
2 tablespoons honey
2 tablespoons unsweetened cocoa powder, plus more to coat
Unsweetened coconut flakes, to coat
Finely chopped almonds, to coat

1. Mix together all the ingredients (except the coconut flakes, almonds, and extra cocoa powder) in a mixing bowl and form into 1-inch balls.

2. Roll each ball in the coconut flakes, almonds, or cocoa powder to make a variety of truffle balls. Place on a serving dish or set aside in an airtight container.

Tip: The hemp seeds add texture to these truffles. If you like a smoother consistency, grind the seeds in a food processor or spice grinder first.

FRESH BERRIES WITH WHIPPED COCONUT CREAM

Lightly sweetened fresh berries with a rich and creamy whipped topping alternative! Low in sugar calories, berries are loaded with protective antioxidants.

SERVES 4

4 cups organic mixed berries (strawberries, raspberries, blueberries, blackberries)
2 teaspoons stevia extract, divided
One 14-ounce can full-fat coconut milk, refrigerated overnight
½ teaspoon vanilla extract

1. Place the berries in a large bowl, sprinkle with 1 teaspoon of the stevia, and refrigerate until ready to serve.

2. Place a medium bowl and the beaters from a mixer in the freezer for 5 minutes.

3. Turn the chilled can of coconut milk upside down and open. Drain off the coconut water and scoop out the solid coconut cream.

4. Mix the coconut cream, remaining 1 teaspoon stevia, and the vanilla in the chilled bowl and beat with the chilled beaters until creamy, about 3 minutes.

5. Divide the mixed berries among four serving dishes and top with the coconut cream.

Tip: The coconut whipped cream does not break down the way dairy cream does. It can be stored for up to 3 days, covered, in the refrigerator.

APPENDIX A
PRE-PROGRAM FOUR-DAY
FOOD/SYMPTOM JOURNAL

The pre-program food journal is meant to make you aware of what you are putting into your body and how you feel on a daily basis before starting the Gut C.A.R.E. Program. Fill out the journal as honestly as you can. No one is going to judge you. Log a Friday through Monday while you are reading and preparing to follow the dietary advice in *Happy Gut*. This way you will capture both your weekday and weekend eating habits. There are spaces for snacks between and after each meal, but only record what you actually do. Simply record how you are eating and feeling before starting the Happy Gut Diet.

Day 1 *Date:* _____   *Symptoms:* _____

Breakfast: _____

Snack: _____

Lunch: _____

Snack: _____

Dinner: _____

Dessert/Snack: _____

Day 2 *Date:* _____ *Symptoms:* _____

Breakfast: _____

Snack: _____

Lunch: _____

Snack: _____

Dinner: _____

Dessert/Snack: _____

Day 3 *Date:* _____ *Symptoms:* _____

Breakfast: _____

Snack: _____

Lunch: _____

Snack: _____

Dinner: _____

Dessert/Snack: _____

Day 4 *Date:* _____ *Symptoms:* _____

Breakfast: _____

Snack: _____

Lunch: _____

Snack: _____

Dinner: _____

Dessert/Snack: _____

APPENDIX B
TWENTY-EIGHT-DAY HAPPY GUT
DIET FOOD/SYMPTOM JOURNAL

You will be measuring your weight and waist circumference once a week, starting with the first day of the twenty-eight-day Gut C.A.R.E. Program. Before you begin recording any measurements, let's go over how to take your weight and waist measurements to ensure consistency in the results.

How to measure your weight: You should measure your weight first thing in the morning with no clothes on. A digital scale will be the most accurate, and you should use the same scale for each weekly measurement for the duration of the program. Don't measure your weight daily, as it may fluctuate and will only add to your anxiety. The big picture and final result are what is important here.

How to measure your waist circumference: This is not the same as the waist size of the clothes you wear, which is measured lower. Find the soft spot on each side of your mid-body in between your lower rib and the top of your pelvic bone (where the "love handles" are). These soft spots are roughly in line with your belly button, but may be an inch above for some people. Measure your waist circumference (in inches or centimeters) at this level without sucking in your abdomen (keep it relaxed). This band represents metabolically active fat—the type that causes inflammation and insulin resistance, leading to the vicious cycle of weight gain and more fat deposition. You should measure your waist in the morning at the same time as you do your weight.

It is important to keep track of your waist circumference and consistently measure it at the same spot, because some weeks will seem slower in terms of weight loss but actually show progress, with a reduction in waist size as you become less bloated and lose stubborn fat from your middle section. Since fat occupies more space but is light compared to muscle and water weight, you may see more movement in your waist circumference than on the scale on some weeks.

To be even more complete in your measurement tracking, you can also keep a log of your biceps circumference (midway between your elbows and shoulders) and thigh circumference (midway between your knees and hips). These measurements will help you keep track of fat loss from these areas as well. You may see losses alternate between the scale and the waist, arms, and thighs.

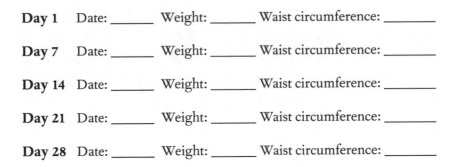

Day 1   Date: _____   Weight: _____   Waist circumference: _____

Day 7   Date: _____   Weight: _____   Waist circumference: _____

Day 14   Date: _____   Weight: _____   Waist circumference: _____

Day 21   Date: _____   Weight: _____   Waist circumference: _____

Day 28   Date: _____   Weight: _____   Waist circumference: _____

For the twenty-eight-day program, every day begins with a gratitude. If you cannot think of a gratitude for a particular day, then use this space to write down a positive affirmation. It serves the same purpose as setting an intention for the day.

TWENTY-EIGHT-DAY HAPPY GUT DIET
FOOD/SYMPTOM JOURNAL

Day 1 *Date:* _____ *Symptoms:* _____
Gratitude: _____

Breakfast Smoothie: _____

Lunch: _____

Snack: _____

Dinner: _____

Snack: _____

Day 2 *Date:* _____ *Symptoms:* _____
Gratitude: _____

Breakfast Smoothie: _____

Lunch: _____

Snack: _____

Dinner: _____

Snack: _____

Day 3 *Date:* _____ *Symptoms:* _____
Gratitude: _____

Breakfast Smoothie: _____

Lunch: _____

Snack: _____

Dinner: _____

Snack: _____

Day 4 *Date:* _____ *Symptoms:* _____
Gratitude: _____

Breakfast Smoothie: _____

Lunch: _____

Snack: _____

Dinner: _____

Snack: _____

Day 5 *Date:* _____ *Symptoms:* _____
Gratitude: _____

Breakfast Smoothie: _____

Lunch: _____

Snack: _____

Dinner: _____

Snack: _____

Day 6 *Date:* _____ *Symptoms:* _____
Gratitude: _____

Breakfast Smoothie: _____

Lunch: _____

Snack: _____

Dinner: _____

Snack: _____

Day 7 *Date:* _____ *Symptoms:* _____
Gratitude: _____

Breakfast Smoothie: _____

Lunch: _____

Snack: _____

Dinner: _____

Snack: _____

Day 8 *Date:* _____ *Symptoms:* _____
Gratitude: _____

Breakfast Smoothie: _____

Lunch: _____

Snack: _____

Dinner: _____

Snack: _____

Day 9 *Date:* _____ *Symptoms:* _____
Gratitude: _____

Breakfast Smoothie: _____

Lunch: _____

Snack: _____

Dinner: _____

Snack: _____

Day 10 *Date:* _____ *Symptoms:* _____
Gratitude: _____

Breakfast Smoothie: _____

Lunch: _____

Snack: _____

Dinner: _____

Snack: _____

Day 11 *Date:* _____ *Symptoms:* _____
Gratitude: _____

Breakfast Smoothie: _____

Lunch: _____

Snack: _____

Dinner: _____

Snack: _____

Day 12 *Date:* _____ *Symptoms:* _____
Gratitude: _____

Breakfast Smoothie: _____

Lunch: _____

Snack: _____

Dinner: _____

Snack: _____

Day 13 *Date:* _____ *Symptoms:* _____
Gratitude: _____

Breakfast Smoothie: _____

Lunch: _____

Snack: _____

Dinner: _____

Snack: _____

Day 14 *Date:* _____ *Symptoms:* _____
Gratitude: _____

Breakfast Smoothie: _____

Lunch: _____

Snack: _____

Dinner: _____

Snack: _____

Day 15 *Date:* _____ *Symptoms:* _____
Gratitude: _____

Breakfast Smoothie: _____

Lunch: _____

Snack: _____

Dinner: _____

Snack: _____

Day 16 *Date:* _____ *Symptoms:* _____
Gratitude: _____

Breakfast Smoothie: _____

Lunch: _____

Snack: _____

Dinner: _____

Snack: _____

Day 17 *Date:* _____ *Symptoms:* _____
Gratitude: _____

Breakfast Smoothie: _____

Lunch: _____

Snack: _____

Dinner: _____

Snack: _____

Day 18 *Date:* _____ *Symptoms:* _____
Gratitude: _____

Breakfast Smoothie: _____

Lunch: _____

Snack: _____

Dinner: _____

Snack: _____

Day 19 *Date:* _____ *Symptoms:* _____
Gratitude: _____

Breakfast Smoothie: _____

Lunch: _____

Snack: _____

Dinner: _____

Snack: _____

Day 20 *Date:* _____ *Symptoms:* _____
Gratitude: _____

Breakfast Smoothie: _____

Lunch: _____

Snack: _____

Dinner: _____

Snack: _____

Day 21 *Date:* _____ *Symptoms:* _____
Gratitude: _____

Breakfast Smoothie: _____

Lunch: _____

Snack: _____

Dinner: _____

Snack: _____

Day 22 *Date:* _____ *Symptoms:* _____
Gratitude: _____

Breakfast Smoothie: _____

Lunch: _____

Snack: _____

Dinner: _____

Snack: _____

Day 23 *Date:* _____ *Symptoms:* _____
Gratitude: _____

Breakfast Smoothie: _____

Lunch: _____

Snack: _____

Dinner: _____

Snack: _____

Day 24 *Date:* _____ *Symptoms:* _____
Gratitude: _____

Breakfast Smoothie: _____

Lunch: _____

Snack: _____

Dinner: _____

Snack: _____

Day 25 *Date:* _____ *Symptoms:* _____
Gratitude: _____

Breakfast Smoothie: _____

Lunch: _____

Snack: _____

Dinner: _____

Snack: _____

Day 26 *Date:* _____ *Symptoms:* _____
Gratitude: _____

Breakfast Smoothie: _____

Lunch: _____

Snack: _____

Dinner: _____

Snack: _____

Day 27 *Date:* _____ *Symptoms:* _____
Gratitude: _____

Breakfast Smoothie: _____

Lunch: _____

Snack: _____

Dinner: _____

Snack: _____

Day 28 *Date:* _____ *Symptoms:* _____
Gratitude: _____

Breakfast Smoothie: _____

Lunch: _____

Snack: _____

Dinner: _____

Snack: _____

CONGRATS! YOU MADE IT!!!

Now take five minutes to complete your *Post-Program Symptoms Questionnaire*.

The Happy Gut Post-Program Symptoms Questionnaire

Rate each of the following symptoms based upon how you feel at the *end* of the Gut C.A.R.E. Program and Happy Gut Diet:

Point Scale

0   *Never* or *almost never* have the symptom

1   *Occasionally* have it, symptom is *not severe*

3   *Occasionally* have it, symptom is *severe*

5   *Frequently* have it, symptom is *not severe*

7   *Frequently* have it, symptom is *severe*

Head

_____ Headaches/migraines

_____ Light-headedness

_____ Dizziness

_____ Insomnia

Total _____

Eyes

_____ Watery, red, or itchy eyes

_____ Swollen or sticky eyelids

_____ Bags or dark circles under eyes

_____ Blurred or tunnel vision (does not include near- or farsightedness)

Total _____

Ears

_____ Itchy ears

_____ Ear infections, earaches

_____ Drainage from ear

_____ Ringing in ears

Total _____

Nose

_____ Nasal congestion

_____ Sinus problems

_____ Runny nose

_____ Sneezing attacks

_____ Excessive mucus production

_____ Frequent colds

Total _____

Mouth/Throat

_____ Chronic cough

_____ Frequently clearing throat of mucus

_____ Sore throat, hoarseness, loss of voice

_____ Swollen, pale, and/or red tongue or gums

_____ White, frothy coating on tongue

_____ Canker sores or mouth ulcers

Total _____

Gut

_____ Nausea, vomiting

_____ Diarrhea

_____ Constipation

_____ Bloated feeling

_____ Excessive belching, passing gas

_____ Heartburn

_____ Abdominal pain

Total _____

Skin

_____ Acne

_____ Hives, rashes, eczema

_____ Hair loss or thinning hair

_____ Flushing, hot flashes

_____ Excessive sweating

Total _____

Chest/Heart

_____ Irregular or skipped heartbeat

_____ Rapid or pounding heartbeat after eating

_____ Chest pain after or in between meals

Total _____

Lungs

_____ Chest tightness or congestion

_____ Asthma, wheezing, or bronchitis

_____ Shortness of breath

_____ Difficulty breathing with exertion

Total _____

Genital/Urinary

_____ Frequent or urgent urination

_____ Difficulty urinating

_____ Penile itching or discharge

_____ Vaginal itching or discharge

Total _____

Joints/Muscle

_____ Painful, swollen, or achy joints

_____ Arthritis

_____ Stiffness or limitation of movement

_____ Painful or achy muscles

_____ Feeling of weakness or fatigue

Total _____

Weight

_____ Excessive eating/drinking

_____ Craving certain foods (like bread or desserts)

_____ Excessive weight gain

_____ Compulsive eating

_____ Water retention

_____ Unexpected weight loss

Total _____

Energy/Activity

_____ Fatigue, sluggishness

_____ Lethargy, hard time finding motivation to move

_____ Excessive energy

_____ Agitation

Total _____

Mind

_____ Memory loss

_____ Confusion, poor comprehension

_____ Mental fog

_____ Poor concentration

_____ Poor balance

_____ Indecisiveness

_____ Word-finding difficulties

_____ Difficulty learning

Total _____

Emotions

_____ Mood swings

_____ Anxiety, fear, nervousness

_____ Anger, irritability, aggressiveness

_____ Depression

Total _____

GRAND TOTAL _____

Compare your post-program individual and total scores with the tallies you recorded in the Pre-Program Symptoms Questionnaire. This is a great way to track your progress. You will clearly see where you have improved as your individual and total scores decrease. It will also help you pinpoint areas that need more attention and will give you a place from which to continue working with your health-care practitioner on symptoms you want to improve.

APPENDIX C
RECOMMENDED SUPPLEMENTS
AND BRANDS

These are some of the highest quality supplements and brands that I trust and use every day with my patients. Many of the nutraceutical companies below only sell through health-care practitioners. It is best that you work with an Integrative or Functional Medicine practitioner, or a naturopath, to guide you on the finest combination of natural products for you. You will find many of the brands I recommend on the Happy Gut website.

Happy Gut and the Gut C.A.R.E. Program
120 East 56th Street, Suite 530
New York, NY 10022
www.happygutlife.com

The statements for each product are for nutritional support. These statements have not been evaluated by the Food & Drug Administration. These products are not intended to diagnose, treat, cure or prevent any diseases.

A resource of information on how to achieve total body wellness through a happy gut. Come join the Happy Gut community, and check out our Happy Gut–approved recipes to continue to inspire you on your path to wellness. You'll also find our recommended products, including individual supplements and the Happy Gut Cleanse to help you achieve gut happiness, cleanse your body, lose weight, gain back your energy, and relieve general body aches and pains.

Gut C.A.R.E. Program supplements:

- **Cleanse Shake**—a hypoallergenic, gluten-free, dairy-free protein powder to help nourish and support gastrointestinal function
- **Cleanse**—supports healthy microbial balance
- **Activate**—a premeal digestive enzyme support
- **Restore**—a high-potency, complete daily probiotic with 100-plus billion CFUs
- **Enhance**—a powder mixture of L-glutamine, DGL, and aloe to support healthy gastrointestinal function
- **Relax**—supports gastrointestinal regularity

Allergy Research Group

2300 North Loop Road
Alameda, CA 94502
(800) 545-9960
www.allergyresearchgroup.com

Originating from the work of Dr. Stephen Levine, Allergy Research Group was one of the first companies to introduce low-allergen products to the market and produces high-quality, hypoallergenic products based on cutting-edge research.

Recommended supplements:

- **FOS Powder**—a prebiotic that supports a healthy intestinal flora
- **GastroCleanse**—supports intestinal regularity
- **Gluten-Gest**—a digestive enzyme combo, which targets difficult-to-digest wheat and gluten peptides (great to use when eating out and not sure if food is completely gluten-free)

Boiron
6 Campus Boulevard
Newtown Square, PA 19073
(800) 264-7661
www.boironusa.com

The active ingredients in homeopathic medicines are micro-doses of plants, animals, and minerals that relieve the same symptoms they cause at full strength (for example, a micro-dose of a coffee bean helps nervousness). Founded in 1932 in France, Boiron, a world leader in homeopathy, maintains the highest standards in manufacturing, complying with U.S. Food and Drug Administration regulations.

Recommended homeopathic remedies:

- **Arsenicum album 30C**—relieves diarrhea from food poisoning
- **Carbo vegetabilis 6C**—relieves bloating and gas in the stomach accompanied by belching
- **Ipecac 30C**—relieves nausea and vomiting
- **Nux vomica 30C**—relieves digestive cramps, especially when associated with overeating

Enzymatic Therapy
825 Challenger Drive
Green Bay, WI 54311
(800) 783-2286
www.enzymatictherapy.com

With a pharmaceutical-minded attention to quality, Enzymatic Therapy is a pioneer in science-based supplements.

Recommended supplements:

- **DGL chew**—a chewable deglycyrrhizinated licorice (DGL) root extract for GI support
- **Peppermint Plus**—an extract of peppermint leaf oil that helps soothe the intestines with its antispasmodic effects; must be taken on an empty stomach

Gaia Herbs
101 Gaia Herbs Drive
Brevard, NC 28712
(800) 831-7780
www.gaiaherbs.com

A brand of herbal remedies known for their purity and integrity to improve patient vitality.

Recommended products:

- **Astragalus Supreme**—supports immune function
- **Kava Kava Root**—supports calm and relaxation
- **Liver Health**—daily support for a healthy liver
- **Para-Shield**—a powerful blend of antiparasitic herbs
- **Sound Sleep**—an herbal formula to facilitate the transition to sleep

Klaire Labs
10439 Double R Boulevard
Reno, NV 89521
(888) 488-2488
www.klaire.com

The mission of Klaire Labs is to provide nutritional support for individuals with severe food allergies and environmental sensitivities. Its probiotics are very high quality, while also being hypoallergenic and dairy- and gluten-free. These products provide support for individuals with dysbiosis, irritable bowel syndrome, inflammatory bowel disease, malabsorption, lactose intolerance, leaky gut syndrome, and food allergies and children with autism spectrum disorders.

Recommended products:

- **Biotagen**—prebiotic support
- **InterFase Plus**—enzyme support
- **Magnesium citrate**—supports bowel regularity
- **Multi-Element Buffered C**—a buffered vitamin C supplement
- **Saccharomyces boulardii**—a great remedy for diarrhea or food poisoning
- **SerenAid**—a multienzyme supplement that helps break down gluten, for instances when you might be exposed (like when eating out)
- **Ther-Biotic Complete**—a complete probiotic
- **Ther-Biotic Complete Powder**—a powder form of the company's broad-spectrum probiotic
- **Ther-Biotic Factor 1**—*Lactobacillus rhamnosus,* proven to reduce inflammation and improve insulin sensitivity
- **Ther-Biotic Factor 4**—four strains of *Bifidobacterium*
- **Ther-Biotic Women's Formula**—a complete probiotic designed for women
- **Vital-Zymes Chewable**—digestive enzyme support

Integrative Therapeutics
825 Challenger Drive
Green Bay, WI 54311
(800) 931-1709
www.integrativepro.com

A brand of nutritional supplements created to combine with diet and lifestyle recommendations for enhanced health.

Recommended products:

- **Berberine Complex**—supports healthy microbial balance
- **Betaine HCl**—supports a healthy stomach pH for protein digestion
- **Cortisol Manager**—supports healthy cortisol levels and restful sleep
- **Glutamine Fortè**—supports a healthy gastrointestinal lining
- **Rhizinate Fructose Free**—chewable deglycyrrhizinated licorice to support a healthy GI mucosa
- **Thymucin**—an astragalus formula for immune support

Metagenics
25 Enterprise
Aliso Viejo, CA 92656
(800) 692-9400
www.metagenics.com

Metagenics has been a long-standing leader in the world of Functional Medicine with supplements that provide consistent results and that are based on the latest science. The company continues to design science-based products and lifestyle medicine programs to create optimal health and wellness. *In collaboration with Metagenics, I have created a special site featuring my favorite products to jump-start you to better gut health. Take advantage of 20 percent off your first order and 10 percent off automatic recurring orders, along with free shipping, at http://happygut.metagenics.com.*

Recommended products:

- **Candibactin-AR**—supports microbial balance
- **Candibactin-BR**—supports microbial balance
- **Glutagenics**—support for a healthy digestive tract lining

- **UltraFlora Balance**—support for a healthy microflora and immune health
- **UltraFlora Integrity**—support for intestinal barrier function
- **UltraFlora Restore**—support for antibiotic-associated diarrhea

Nordic Naturals

111 Jennings Drive
Watsonville, CA 95076
(800) 662-2544
www.nordicnaturals.com

A company born in Arctic Norway, Nordic Naturals has become a leading supplier of high-quality fish oils worldwide. Its products support heart health and the natural anti-inflammatory response.

Recommended products:

- **ProDHA**—supports a healthy mood and cognitive function
- **ProEPA with Concentrated GLA**—an excellent anti-inflammatory combination
- **ProEPA Xtra**—the highest potency EPA concentrate, supports immunity and healthy inflammatory levels
- **ProOmega**—the company's most popular omega-3 formulation

Pure Encapsulations

490 Boston Post Road
Sudbury, MA 01776
(800) 753-2277
www.pureencapsulations.com

A line of research-based, hypoallergenic nutritional supplements in easy-to-swallow capsules that are devoid of hidden fillers, coatings, artificial colors, or other excipients.

Recommended products:

- **Betaine HCl Pepsin**—promotes healthy digestion in the stomach
- **Caprylic acid**—support for a healthy *Candida* balance
- **DGL Plus**—herbal support for the GI tract
- **Digestion GB**—digestive enzyme support with extra support for fat digestion
- **Digestive Enzymes Ultra**—a comprehensive blend of vegetarian digestive enzymes
- **G.I. Fortify**—supports all key aspects of digestive function
- **L-glutamine powder**—supports the mucosal lining of the GI tract
- **Liver-G.I. Detox**—support for liver and gastrointestinal detoxification
- **Metabolic Xtra**—supports insulin function and glucose metabolism
- **MicroDefense**—a combination of antimicrobial/antiparasitic herbs
- **MotilCalm**—provides calming and immune support for the GI tract
- **MotilPro**—supports healthy gut motility
- **Pancreatic Enzyme Formula**—designed to aid in the body's natural digestive process
- **Peptic-Care ZC**—a zinc carnosine formula for optimal stomach health
- **Probiotic 50B**—a potent probiotic with 50 billion CFU per capsule
- **Vitamin D$_3$**—1,000 IU, 5,000 IU, and 10,000 IU formulations

Thorne Research
25820 Highway 2 West
Sandpoint, ID 83864
(800) 228-1966
www.thorne.com

Thorne Research is dedicated to providing superior dietary supplements of the highest quality and purity to improve overall patient health.

Recommended supplements:

- **Bio-Gest**—a comprehensive blend of digestive enzymes
- **FiberMend**—soluble fiber formula to help maintain regularity
- **FloraMend Prime Probiotic**—stomach-acid resistant probiotic blend for gastrointestinal health
- **MediClear Plus**—hypoallergenic pea/rice protein powder that supports liver detoxification and the body's anti-inflammatory response
- **Perma-Clear**—intestinal permeability support
- **Plantizyme**—a plant-based enzyme formula

Vital Nutrients
45 Kenneth Dooley Drive
Middletown, CT 06457
(888) 328-9992
www.vitalnutrients.net

Vital Nutrients is recognized as *The Leader in Quality Assurance* in the professional supplement industry with more than two hundred pharmaceutical-grade supplements for overall health and well-being. All of the company's products are extensively tested for authenticity, potency, and environmental contaminants. *To take advantage of a special Happy Gut offer and receive* **10 percent off** *all Vital Nutrients products, register on the Vital Nutrients website and use* **practitioner code 0747.**

Recommended products:

- *Acidophilus/Bifidobacter/FOS*—pre- and probiotic support, promotes healthy digestion; dairy-free formula
- **BCQ**—the company's best-selling product; supports a healthy inflammatory response for joint, sinus, and digestive health
- **Berberine**—supports healthy microbial balance and healthy blood sugar levels

- **Betaine HCl Pepsin and Gentian Root Extract**—powerful digestive support for the stomach
- **DGL powder**—promotes healthy GI mucus secretion and provides nutritional support for the stomach
- **GI Repair Powder***—helps support healthy GI function, supports collagen repair, and maintains healthy intestinal permeability
- **Glutamine powder**—supports healthy GI tract function and immune support
- **Heartburn Tx**—relief for occasional heartburn and indigestion
- **Pancreatic enzymes**—digestive enzymes support
- **Slippery elm bark powder**—promotes mucus production in the GI tract lining to allow for the easy movement of food and to support bowel movements
- **Whole Fiber Fusion**—natural source of dietary fiber composed of whole plants and seeds; relieves occasional constipation

*Contains crustacean fish: lobster, crab, and/or shrimp. Contains milk: lactoferrin is derived from New Zealand cow's milk.

Xymogen
6900 Kingspointe Parkway
Orlando, FL 32819
(800) 647-6100
www.xymogen.com

A family-owned company that calls on the most talented professionals in medicine, nutrition, and dietary supplements to develop formulas using the latest science and research.

Recommended products:

- **Berbemycin**—supports microbial balance
- **Candicidal**—natural support for a balanced GI system with anti-yeast herbs
- **ColonX**—support for intestinal regularity
- **GlutAloeMine**—enhanced gastrointestinal support for healthy GI function
- **L-glutamine powder**—for GI mucosal lining support
- **ProbioMax Daily DF**—probiotic with 30 billion CFU per capsule
- **ProbioMax DF**—probiotic with 100 billion CFU per capsule

APPENDIX D
RESOURCES

FINDING A FUNCTIONAL MEDICINE PRACTITIONER

The Institute for Functional Medicine
505 South 336th Street, Suite 600
Federal Way, WA 98003
(800) 228-0622
www.functionalmedicine.org

Search for a Functional Medicine practitioner near you by zip code using the "Find a Practitioner" link on the home page.

Cell Science Systems
Alcat Worldwide
852 South Military Trail
Deerfield Beach, FL 33442
(800) 872-5228
www.alcat.com

The ALCAT test is considered the gold standard for identifying non-IgE-mediated reactions to foods, chemicals, and other substances. Testing options include the ALCAT Food and Chemical Sensitivity Test, a Gut Health Profile, and other specialized tests.

Recommended panels:

• Comprehensive Wellness 3, 4, 5, or 6—each panel measures a
  different quantity of foods, food additives, mold, and other substances
• Platinum Comprehensive

Commonwealth Laboratories, Inc.
39 Norman Street
Salem, MA 01970
(978) 599-1380
www.hydrogenbreathtesting.com

Hydrogen and methane breath analysis from Commonwealth Labs provides a fast, reliable, and convenient diagnostic tool for identifying small intestinal bacterial overgrowth (SIBO), a leading cause of the symptoms associated with irritable bowel syndrome (IBS), as well as other digestive disorders, including lactose intolerance, fructose intolerance, sucrose intolerance, and *Helicobacter pylori* stomach infection.

Recommended breath tests:

- SIBO
- Lactose intolerance/lactose malabsorption
- Fructose intolerance/fructose malabsorption
- *Helicobacter pylori*

Cyrex Laboratories

5040 North 15th Avenue, Suite 307
Phoenix, AZ 85015
(877) 772-9739
www.cyrexlabs.com

A laboratory specializing in immunology and autoimmunity that offers antibody testing for the early detection and monitoring of complex autoimmune conditions such as celiac disease.

Recommended profiles:

- Array 3—Wheat/Gluten Proteome Reactivity and Autoimmunity
- Array 4—Gluten-Associated Cross-Reactive Foods and Foods Sensitivity
- Array 5—Multiple Autoimmune Reactivity Screen

Diagnos-Techs Clinical and Research Laboratory

19110 66th Avenue S, Building G
Kent, WA 98032
(800) 878-3787
www.diagnostechs.com

Test panel options include an Adrenal Stress Index Panel, a Female Hormone Panel, a Food Allergy (Sensitivity) Panel, a Gastrointestinal Health Panel, a Male Hormone Panel, and a Menopausal Hormone Panel.

Doctor's Data
3755 Illinois Avenue
St. Charles, IL 60174
(800) 323-2784
www.doctorsdata.com

A multitude of tests are offered under the categories of clinical microbiology, toxic and essential elements, nutritional, environmental exposure and detoxification, and cardiovascular testing.

Recommended panels:

• Comprehensive Stool Analysis with Parasitology
• Intestinal Permeability

Dunwoody Labs
9 Dunwoody Park, Suite 121
Dunwoody, GA 30338
(678) 736-6374
www.dunwoodylabs.com

Provides unique food-sensitivity testing using a food allergy profile that detects delayed allergic responses, including immune complex formation, for a higher sensitivity than other panels.

Recommended panels:

• C3d Food Sensitivity
• Gut Triad
• Stool Culture

ELISA/ACT Biotechnologies

109 Carpenter Drive, Suite 100
Sterling, VA 20164
(800) 553-5472
www.elisaact.com

The LRA by ELISA/ACT test is an alternative to IgG testing for patients with gluten reactivity as it is the only test that measures the three types of delayed sensitivity reactions of reactive antibodies (IgA, IgM, and IgG), immune complexes, and T-cell direct activation.

EnteroLab

13657 Jupiter Road, Suite 106
Dallas, TX 75238
(972) 686-6689
www.enterolab.com

Screening tests for gluten sensitivity and other antigenic food sensitivities.

Genova Diagnostics

63 Zillicoa Street
Asheville, NC 28801
(800) 522-4762
www.gdx.net

Genova provides a variety of tests to help diagnose underlying gut issues. Recommended panels:

- Anti-*Candida* Antibody
- Bacterial Overgrowth of the Small Intestine

- Comprehensive Digestive Stool Analysis 2.0
- Comprehensive Parasitology Profile
- Fat-Soluble Vitamins Profile
- GI Effects Comprehensive Profile—Stool
- GI Effects Microbial Ecology Profile
- *Helicobacter pylori* Stool Antigen EIA
- Intestinal Permeability Assessment
- Lactose Intolerance Breath Test
- Organix Dysbiosis Profile—Urine

Great Plains Laboratory

11813 West 77th Street

Lenexa, KS 66214

(800) 288-0383

www.greatplainslaboratory.com

Testing options include Full Organic Acids Test, IgG Food Allergy Test with *Candida*, Comprehensive Stool Analysis, and Gluten/Casein Peptides Test.

Meridian Valley Lab

6839 Fort Dent Way, Suite 206

Tukwila, WA 98188

(855) 405-8378

www.meridianvalleylab.com

Allergy and hormone testing, specializing in comprehensive urine, hormone, and metabolite testing.

Recommended panels:

- E-95 Basic Food Panel
- A-95 Extended Food Panel

U.S. Bio Tek Laboratories
16020 Linden Avenue
North Shoreline, WA 98133
(206) 365-1256
www.usbiotek.com

State-of-the-art testing, including:

- *Candida* Antibodies and Antigen Panel
- Celiac Antibody Panel
- Comprehensive Urinary Metabolic Profile
- Comprehensive Urinary Steroid Hormone Profile
- Environmental Pollutants Profile
- IgE/IgG/IgA Antibody Assessment Testing

FROM THE OCEAN AND PASTURES TO THE KITCHEN

Alderspring Ranch
www.alderspring.com
A supplier of certified organic, pasture-raised, grass-fed beef from the mountains of Idaho. Cattle are raised on hay without grain of any kind.

NorthStar Bison
www.northstarbison.com
A family-run ranch in northwest Wisconsin and east central Minnesota, supplying antibiotic- and hormone-free, pasture-raised meats, including bison, beef, lamb, elk, chicken, and ostrich.

Pure Indian Foods
www.pureindianfoods.com

A selection of grass-fed, organic cultured ghee and spiced ghee; Indian spices; and teas, as well as other Indian delights.

Vital Choice: Wild Seafood and Organics

Go to www.vitalchoice.com/happygut for 10 percent off your first order.

A great selection of wild-caught cold-water fish from flash-frozen wild salmon to canned salmon, low-mercury tuna, sardines, and other organic choices.

360 Cookware

www.360cookware.com

Use promo code "getahappygut" for 10 percent off your orders.

360 Cookware is stainless steel–coated cooking ware with a core of bonded aluminum that creates remarkable heat conductivity. With its unique 360 Vapor Cooking technology, food can be cooked with less oil, less water, and at lower temperatures to preserve the greatest amount of nutrients and flavor while making healthier, greener dishes for the whole family.

RECOMMENDED READING AND DOCUMENTARIES

Books

The Blood Sugar Solution: The UltraHealthy Program for Losing Weight, Preventing Disease, and Feeling Great Now! by Dr. Mark Hyman. www.bloodsugarsolution.com
Dr. Mark Hyman reveals that the secret to weight loss and the prevention of diabetes, heart disease, stroke, dementia, and cancer is maintaining balanced insulin levels.

The Blood Sugar Solution 10-Day Detox Diet: Activate Your Body's Natural Ability to Burn Fat and Lose Weight Fast by Dr. Mark Hyman
www.10daydetox.com/successfuldetox
A weight-loss program designed by Dr. Mark Hyman, whose key to losing and maintaining weight is keeping a low insulin level.

The Body Ecology Diet: Recovering Your Health and Rebuilding Your Immunity by Donna Gates
www.bodyecology.com
The book focuses on *Candida* and yeast overgrowth and how to heal the gut using cultured foods.

Breaking the Vicious Cycle: Intestinal Health Through Diet by Elaine Gloria Gottschall
www.breakingtheviciouscycle.info
A guide to the Specific Carbohydrate Diet, which is highly effective in helping to heal inflammatory bowel disease.

The Cancer-Fighting Kitchen: Nourishing Big-Flavor Recipes for Cancer Treatment and Recovery by Rebecca Katz
www.rebeccakatz.com/the-cancer-fighting-kitchen
Features 150 science-based, nutrient-rich recipes that are designed to stimulate appetite and address cancer treatment side effects such as fatigue, nausea, dehydration, and more.

Clean Gut: The Breakthrough Plan for Eliminating the Root Cause of Disease and Revolutionizing Your Health by Dr. Alejandro Junger
www.cleanprogram.com
Offers an alternative to treating symptoms as they arise by preemptively attacking diseases before they appear through a cleansing program.

Crazy Sexy Diet: Eat Your Veggies, Ignite Your Spark, and Live Like You Mean It! by Kris Carr
www.kriscarr.com/products/crazy-sexy-diet
Kris Carr is a cancer survivor who shares her low-sugar, vegetarian program for healing the body.

Food Rules: An Eater's Manual by Michael Pollan
www.michaelpollan.com/books/food-rules
After years of extensive research into where our food comes from and how it's produced, Michael Pollan, a leading food writer, explains his philosophy of eating. These are simple food guidelines to eat in the healthiest way possible.

Grain Brain: The Surprising Truth About Wheat, Carbs, and Sugar—Your Brain's Silent Killers by Dr. David Perlmutter
www.drperlmutter.com/about/grain-brain-by-david-perlmutter
Renowned neurologist Dr. David Perlmutter discusses the destructive nature of both healthy and unhealthy carbs on the brain.

Peace Is Every Breath: A Practice for Our Busy Lives by Thich Nhat Hanh
Holy man and Buddhist leader Thich Nhat Hanh shows how each and every one of us can experience inner peace and happiness by practicing mindfulness in the simplest of moments in our daily lives.

Peace Is Every Step: The Path of Mindfulness in Everyday Life by Thich Nhat Hanh
World-renowned Zen master and spiritual leader Thich Nhat Hanh teaches how to find peace within all life circumstances—especially the ones that stress us out the most.

The Power of Now: A Guide to Spiritual Enlightenment by Eckhart Tolle
www.eckharttolle.com/books/now
A guide to spiritual enlightenment that depicts the reader as a creator of his or her own pain and explains how to live a pain-free identity.

It Starts with Food: Discover the Whole30 and Change Your Life in Unexpected Ways by Melissa Hartwig and Dallas Hartwig
www.whole9life.com/itstartswithfood
Outlines a balanced and sustainable eating plan to improve one's lifestyle.

Wheat Belly: Lose the Wheat, Lose the Weight, and Find Your Path Back to Health by Dr. William Davis
www.wheatbelly.com
Dr. William Davis explains that excess fat is due to the adverse health effects from a daily intake of wheat.

Documentaries
Fed Up
www.fedupmovie.com
How America's obesity epidemic is linked to our overconsumption of sugar, and the food industry's role in exacerbating it.

Food, Inc.
www.takepart.com/foodinc
A look at America's corporate-controlled food industry by writers
Robert Kenner, Elise Pearlstein, and Kim Roberts.

Food Matters
www.foodmatters.tv
An examination by nutritionists, naturopaths, doctors, and journalists of
how the food we eat can either help or hurt our health.

Forks Over Knives
www.forksoverknives.com
An investigation of the claim that most, if not all, of the degenerative
diseases that affect the population can be controlled, or reversed, by
discarding our present menu of animal-based, processed foods, by
writer and director Lee Fulkerson.

King Corn
www.kingcorn.net
A documentary about two friends at an East Coast college who move
west to learn where their food comes from, by writers Aaron Woolf, Ian
Cheney, Curtis Ellis, and Jeffrey K. Miller.

Super Size Me
Morgan Spurlock personally explores the penalties on his health of
eating a diet of food exclusively from McDonald's for one month to
assess the impact of the fast-food industry on our health.

WEBSITES

Happy Gut and the Gut C.A.R.E. Program
www.happygutlife.com
A resource full of tips for living with a happy gut, including recipes and products to help you support gut health.

Ecomii Blog: The Food and Health Alternative
www.ecomii.com/blogs/food
An alternative approach to health, wellness, and disease prevention. Editor Marie Oser and her team of bloggers bring you creative, natural solutions to issues affecting your health and well-being.

Environmental Working Group's Dirty Dozen and Clean Fifteen
www.ewg.org/foodnews
A guide for shoppers to avoid pesticide-coated produce.

Environmental Working Group's Food Scores
www.ewg.org/foodscores
A guide to eating right based on a scoring of nutrition, ingredient concerns, and degree of processing.

Kris Carr
www.kriscarr.com
The blog and wellness shop of the *New York Times* and Amazon number one best-selling author on wellness.

Mark's Daily Apple

www.marksdailyapple.com

Mark Sisson's daily blog on health, nutrition, fitness, the health industry, and his low-carb, Paleo, primal lifestyle.

MindBodyGreen

www.mindbodygreen.com

Videos and articles on the mind and body, as well as organic lifestyle tips.

Rebecca Katz

www.rebeccakatz.com

Books, videos, recipes, and more from Rebecca Katz, a nationally recognized culinary translator.

Exposure to environmental toxins, especially those in sunscreens and skin creams, should be eliminated for overall body wellness. For reducing your exposure to topical toxins that accumulate in your body fat and cause weight gain, see:

Environmental Working Group's Safer Sunscreen Guide

www.ewg.org/2015sunscreen

The EWG's 2015 *Guide to Safer Sunscreens*.

Environmental Working Group's Skin Deep Cosmetics Database

www.ewg.org/skindeep

The Skin Deep database supplies practical solutions to protect oneself from everyday exposures to chemicals.

APPENDIX E
GUT-RELATED MEDICATION
SIDE EFFECTS

People often assume if something is a medicine, it will help them, but they discount the seriousness of potential side effects of such common drugs like Advil or Aleve. Below is a list of symptoms and some of the common over-the-counter (OTC) medications that can cause them.

SYMPTOMS	COMMON OTC MEDICINAL CULPRITS
Abdominal pain/bloating	Antibiotics (like Augmentin, Zithromax, Clindamycin)
Constipation	Codeine, pain medications (like Vicodin, Percocet, Hydrocodone, Oxycontin, Tylenol #3), cough syrup with codeine, antidiarrheals (Imodium, Lomotil)
Diarrhea	Oral contrast (barium), senna, psyllium husks, antibiotics (like Augmentin, Zithromax, Clindamycin), Lactulose

SYMPTOMS	COMMON OTC MEDICINAL CULPRITS
Gastrointestinal bleeding or ulcers	Nonsteroidal anti-inflammatories, or NSAIDs (like Advil, Aleve, ibuprofen, aspirin)
Leaky gut syndrome (hyperpermeability)	Nonsteroidal anti-inflammatories, or NSAIDs (like Advil, Aleve, ibuprofen, aspirin), antibiotics
Nausea	Antibiotics (especially Doxycycline, Augmentin)

ACKNOWLEDGMENTS

I have so many people to thank—all the helpers, teachers, and guides I have met along the way as this path was paved. There were guides who inspired. There were teachers who challenged, helpers who came and went for but a brief moment, and those who joined me on the trek. It would be impossible to thank every single person. Although I didn't know it at the time, this journey really began in high school, where I initially learned how to string together the written word into well-thought-out prose in my English and literature classes. And later on where, as a blog contributor to Ecomii.com's Food and Health Blog (edited so meticulously by Marie Oser), I learned how to make science understandable and concise.

To the Institute for Functional Medicine: thank you for inspiring me to reconnect with why I became a doctor in the first place. I believe true medicine lies in uncovering the root causes of illness, and it is through your incredible faculty that I have learned how to apply the science of Functional Medicine to the care of my patients. I am indebted to a courageous group of doctors and scientists, including Jeffrey Bland, Dr. Mark Hyman, Dr. David Perlmutter, Dr. Frank Lipman, Dr. Alejandro Junger, and Dr. William David, who believed they could—and have—changed the face of medicine.

Anyone who has written a book knows it is a long journey to get to the point where you can put the stamp of approval on a manuscript. Along the way, you experience sweat, tears, rewriting, reworking, and the back-to-the-drawing-board feeling, until, as if through the help of multiple sculptors chiseling away at a rock, one day the book takes form and assumes a life of its own. Candace Johnson of Change It Up Editing was my unwavering companion through this entire process. From the very first moment we met over the phone, I had a "gut feeling" you were the one to work with. No matter how many times we had to rewrite or reorganize the book, you were always there for me with a positive attitude that kept me going. Your editorial input was invaluable from the early stages of my book proposal to the writing of the book. And I am indebted to you for christening the book with the name that everyone loved—"Happy Gut."

Thank you to my literary agent, Stephany Evans, president of Fine Print Literary Management, for hitting reply on that faith-filled e-mail I sent you in late December 2012 when I was looking for an agent. I knew I needed someone to help me navigate the book world and guide me on shaping my idea into a winning proposal. You gave me one of the greatest gifts one can give an emerging writer—you believed in me, and that faith pushed me forward to find the inner strength I needed, while taking care of patients full time, to work on refining my original proposal. As the manuscript evolved, your input was vital to the creation of a work we can all feel proud of.

To Lisa Sharkey, director of creative development at HarperCollins, I am thrilled to finally work with you. I don't believe in coincidences— our fateful meeting that spring day in 2006 was what opened the door to and launched me on this path. As you have reminded me, I told you I wanted to write a book the very first day I met you. Well, here we are! Thank you for all the wisdom you have shared throughout the years and for always pushing me to be a better doctor and person.

To Amy Bendell, my unfaltering editor: although the words and content of the book are a result of my endless hours of research, conferences, and clinical experience, it is through your skilled editorial eye that we forged this into an easy-to-understand guide to the gut and so much more. Thank you for having the patience to work with an at times stubborn, but moldable, first-time author. After many editing rounds, it was a sigh of relief and an internal jump for joy to hear you say, "This chapter is ready for publishing." I learned so much from you about how to present information in "digestible bites" (pun intended).

Thank you to the incredible team at William Morrow, which has been excited about and championed this book from our very first meeting. Thanks to Mumtaz Mustafa: your incredible graphic design skills created a beautiful book cover we all loved from the very beginning. Thanks also to Alieza Schvimer for coordinating all communications and making sure that we stayed on time with production. Thanks to all the individuals who worked in the background to make this book possible. It has been a pleasure to work with such an enthusiastic, committed, and professional group of people.

Thank you to my yoga teachers, Paula Tursi and Janet Dailey Butler: your wisdom and shared experience made Chapter 8, "The Body-Gut Connection," possible. Although I helped tie in the information you present to the science behind it and to my program for healing the gut, it is primarily your voices that built this invaluable chapter. I have loved yoga and meditation from my initial introduction to them in 1995. It is a joy to include your yoga postures, breathing exercises, and meditation for gut health and total body wellness. I believe in a 360-degree approach to health, and this chapter helps round out the dietary and supplement guidelines I give the reader.

To nutritionist and chef Marlisa Brown and chef Mikaela Reuben, thank you for your time and commitment in creating the mouthwatering, delicious recipes that complement my dietary guidelines for a *happy gut*. You helped bring the words to the table with inspired smoothies, entreés, salads, side dishes, and even *Happy Gut*–approved desserts.

To Jade Dressler, my branding and social media consultant, thank you for your indefatigable dedication to the "why"—the meaning behind everything I do. I trust you wholeheartedly with my vision. You have been the steady hand that has listened patiently, advised, co-created, and inspired me to dream bigger.

To Ryan Gibboney, my talented graphic designer, thank you for helping me create the clear, easy-to-understand diagrams that explain in pictures what I say in words. And Michelle Kauffman, my research assistant, who was a great source of ancillary support.

To Digital Natives, my savvy web-design team responsible for translating our vision into a living, breathing, user-friendly website where Happy Gut—the book, the brand, and so much more—have come to life.

To the team at *Pedre Integrative Health* for your untiring dedication to helping our patients achieve their wellness goals.

To my partner, Tanyette Colon: you taught me to be steadfast and never give up, regardless of the road blocks in life. Thank you for being the mirror I could bounce my ideas off of, and for being the first to believe that a book about the gut was the one I should commit to.

I also have to mention my sisters, Lisette and Laura, for being unflappable sounding boards and sources of encouragement.

And finally, my son, Ambrose, thank you for being a source of light and joy. You make it all worthwhile.

There are many more I wish I could mention; know that you live with gratitude in my heart.

Last but not least, I am forever grateful to all my patients: you have been as much my teachers as I have been yours. Thank you for your trust and for the opportunity to work with each and every one of you. This book is for you and for all the patients I may never get a chance to work with directly. My desire is to inspire you on the path to healthier living through a healthy gut.

NOTES

Part I: It's All About the Gut
Chapter 1: It's All in Your Gut

1. Babies born via C-section do not benefit from this initial colonization but can still acquire helpful bacteria through breast-feeding.

2. The Cleveland Clinic, a nationally recognized center of health-care excellence, has realized this by creating a Center for Functional Medicine, directed by Dr. Mark Hyman, to work in tandem with its excellent doctors.

3. Ridaura, V. K., et al. "Gut Microbiota from Twins Discordant for Obesity Modulate Metabolism in Mice." *Science* 341, no. 6150 (Sept. 2013): doi: 10.1126/science.1241214.

4. Vrieze, A., et al. "Transfer of Intestinal Microbiota from Lean Donors Increases Insulin Sensitivity in Individuals with Metabolic Syndrome." *Gastroenterology* 143, no. 4 (Oct. 2012): 913–6.

5. Itzkowitz, S. H., and X. Yio. "Inflammation and Cancer IV. Colorectal Cancer in Inflammatory Bowel Disease: The Role of Inflammation." *American Journal of Physiology: Gastrointestinal and Liver Physiology* 287 (July 2004): G7–17.

6. O'Byrne, K. J., and A. G. Dalgleish. "Chronic Immune Activation and Inflammation as the Cause of Malignancy." *British Journal of Cancer* 85, no. 4 (Aug. 2001): 473–83.

7. International Agency for Research on Cancer. "GLOBOCAN 2012: Estimated Cancer Incidence, Mortality and Prevalence Worldwide in 2012." World Health

Organization, accessed Sept. 27, 2014, http://globocan.iarc.fr/Pages/fact_sheets_cancer.aspx.

8. Chen, X., and C. S. Yang. "Esophageal Adenocarcinoma: A Review and Perspectives on the Mechanism of Carcinogenesis and Chemoprevention." *Carcinogenesis* 22, no. 8 (Aug. 2001): 1119–29.

9. Itzkowitz and Yio, "Inflammation and Cancer IV."

10. Higaki, S., et al. "Metaplastic Polyp of the Colon Develops in Response to Inflammation." *Journal of Gastroenterology and Hepatology* 14, no. 7 (July 1999): 709–714.

11. Rao, V. P., et al. "Breast Cancer: Should Gastrointestinal Bacteria Be on Our Radar Screen?" *Cancer Research* 67, no. 3 (Feb. 2007): 847–50.

12. Rudwaleit, M., and D. Baeten. "Ankylosing Spondylitis and Bowel Disease." *Best Practice and Research: Clinical Rheumatology* 20, no. 3 (June 2006): 451–71.

Chapter 2: The Happy Gut Diet: Phase I Explained

1. Lenoir, M., et al. "Intense Sweetness Surpasses Cocaine Reward." *PLOS ONE* (Aug. 1, 2007): doi: 10.1371/journal.pone.0000698.

2. Fowler, S. P. "Diet Soft Drink Consumption Is Associated with Increased Incidence of Overweight and Obesity in the San Antonio Heart Study." Paper presented at the Sixty-Fifth Scientific Sessions of the American Diabetes Association, San Diego, CA, June 10–14, 2005.

3. Gardener, H., et al. "Diet Soft Drink Consumption Is Associated with an Increased Risk of Vascular Events in the Northern Manhattan Study." *Journal of General Internal Medicine* 27, no. 9 (Sept. 2012): 1120–6.

4. Teschemacher, H. "Opioid Receptor Ligands Derived from Food Proteins." *Current Pharmaceutical Design* 9, no. 16 (2003): 1331–44.

5. Most commercial oat brands, including oat bran and oat syrup, may be contaminated with gluten because they are often processed in plants that also process gluten-containing grains. Gluten-free oats are available in health-food stores; however, some people with gluten sensitivity can sometimes be sensitive to a similar protein found in oats. When eliminating gluten-containing grains from the diet, it is important to pay attention to this in case you are one of those people who also react to oats.

6. "What Triggers Autoimmunity?" *Lancet* 2, no. 8446 (July 1985): 78–9.

7. Glycemic index is a number given to foods that indicates the degree to which

that food will raise a person's blood glucose. The numbers typically range from 50 to 100, where 100 represents the effect of pure glucose. Foods with high glycemic index scores (close to 100) will raise the blood sugar more, leading to all we have discussed about insulin resistance and weight gain.

8. Cabrera-Chávez, F., et al. "Maize Prolamins Resistant to Peptic-Tryptic Digestion Maintain Immune-Recognition by IgA from Some Celiac Disease Patients." *Plant Foods for Human Nutrition* 67, no. 1 (Mar. 2012): 24, 30.

9. Campbell, T. Colin, with Thomas M. Campbell II. *The China Study: The Most Comprehensive Study of Nutrition Ever Conducted and the Startling Implications for Diet, Weight Loss and Long-Term Health.* Dallas, TX: BenBella Books, 2005, p. 209.

10. Roundup is the trade name of a glyphosate herbicide developed by the Monsanto Corporation to kills weeds that compete with commercial crops grown around the globe.

11. Avoid nightshades if you have an inflammatory, pain, autoimmune, or arthritic disorder. Otherwise, nightshades are allowed in limited quantities.

12. Ghee is a form of clarified butter that originated in India. It is prepared by simmering butter at low heat and removing the residue that rises to the top. This residue contains all the proteins that cause dairy sensitivities. Thus, by removing these proteins, even individuals with a dairy sensitivity can have ghee, and it can be very healing for the gut. See recipes containing ghee in Chapter 9.

13. A recipe for Homemade Almond Milk is included in Chapter 9. The benefit of a homemade nut milk is that it will be free of preservatives and thickeners, like carrageenan.

14. See Chapter 3 for more details.

15. Some people have a sensitivity to xylitol (commonly found in sugar-free gums) and should avoid it as well.

Part II: The Gut C.A.R.E. Program: Twenty-Eight Days to a New You
Chapter 3: Eliminate Symptoms and Maintain Your Health with the Gut C.A.R.E. Program

1. Sicherer, S. H. "Manifestations of Food Allergy: Evaluation and Management." *American Family Physician* 59, no. 2 (Jan. 1999): 415–24.

2. Edwards, M. "Fetal Death and Reduced Birth Rates Associated with Exposure to Lead-Contaminated Drinking Water." *Environmental Science and Technology* 48, no. 1 (2014): 739–46.

3. Hao, J., et al. "Reduction of Pesticide Residues on Fresh Vegetables with Electrolyzed Water Treatment." *Journal of Food Science* 76, no. 4 (May 2011): C520–4.

4. Environmental Working Group. "The Pollution in Newborns: A Benchmark Investigation of Industrial Chemicals, Pollutants and Pesticides in Umbilical Cord Blood," posted July 14, 2005, http://www.ewg.org/research/body-burden -pollution-newborns.

5. Harman, Greg. "New Federal Data Shows Autism Rates Are Booming. Local Researchers Are Finding Industrial Chemicals May Play a Role." *San Antonio Current*, May 2, 2012.

6. De Tata, V. "Association of Dioxin and Other Persistent Organic Pollutants (POPs) with Diabetes: Epidemiological Evidence and New Mechanisms of Beta Cell Dysfunction." *International Journal of Moleuclar Science* 15, no. 5 (May 2014): 7787–811.

7. Bavishi, C., and H. L. Dupont. "Systematic Review: The Use of Proton Pump Inhibitors and Increased Susceptibility to Enteric Infection." *Alimentary Pharmacology and Therapeutics* 34, nos. 11–12 (Dec. 2011): 1269–81.

8. Cho, C. H. "Zinc: Absorption and Role in Gastrointestinal Metabolism and Disorders." *Digestive Diseases* 9, no. 1 (1991): 49–60.

9. Silva, M., et al. "Antimicrobial Substance from a Human *Lactobacillus* Strain." *Antimicrobial Agents and Chemotherapy* 31, no. 8 (Aug. 1987): 1231–3.

10. Malin, M., et al. "Promotion of IgA Immune Response in Patients with Crohn's Disease by Oral Bacteriotherapy with *Lactobacillus GG*." *Annals of Nutrition and Metabolism* 40, no. 3 (1996): 137–45.

11. Roos, K., and S. Holm. "The Use of Probiotics in Head and Neck Infections." *Current Infectious Disease Reports* 4, no. 3 (2002): 211–6.

12. Roos, K., E. G. Håkansson, and S. Holm. "Effect of Recolonisation with 'Interfering' Alpha *Streptococci* on Recurrences of Acute and Secretory Otitis Media in Children: Randomised Placebo Controlled Trial." *British Medical Journal* 322, no. 7280 (2001): 210–2.

13. If dairy based, only after the twenty-eight-day Happy Gut Diet. See Chapter 5.

14. Rembacken, B. J., et al. "Non-Pathogenic *Escherichia coli* Versus Mesalazine for the Treatment of Ulcerative Colitis: A Randomised Trial." *Lancet* 354, no. 9179 (Aug. 1999): 635–9.

15. Guslandi, M., et al. "*Saccharomyces boulardii* in Maintenance Treatment of Crohn's Disease." *Digestive Diseases and Sciences* 45, no. 7 (July 2000): 1462–4.

16. Klimberg, V. S., et al. "Oral Glutamine Accelerates Healing of the Small

Intestine and Improves Outcome After Whole Abdominal Radiation." *Archives of Surgery* 125, no. 8 (Aug. 1990): 1040–5.

17. Krausse, R., et al. "In Vitro Anti–*Helicobacter pylori* Activity of Extractum Liquiritiae, Glycyrrhizin and Its Metabolites." *Journal of Antimicrobial Chemotherapy* 54, no. 1 (July 2004): 243–6.

18. Fiore, C., et al. "A History of the Therapeutic Use of Liquorice in Europe." *Journal of Ethnopharmacology* 99, no. 3 (July 2005): 317–24.

19. Ming, L. J., and A. C. Yin. "Therapeutic Effects of Glycyrrhizic Acid." *Natural Product Communications* 8, no. 3 (Mar. 2013): 415–8.

20. Reuter, J., I. Merfort, and C. M. Schempp. "Botanicals in Dermatology: An Evidence-Based Review." *American Journal of Clinical Dermatology* 11, no. 4 (2010): 247–67.

21. Lee, C. H., et al. "Protective Mechanism of Glycyrrhizin on Acute Liver Injury Induced by Carbon Tetrachloride in Mice." *Biological and Pharmaceutical Bulletin* 30, no. 10 (Oct. 2007): 1898–904.

22. Zhang, Y., et al. "Effects of Glycyrrhizin on Blood Pressure and Its Mechanisms." *Zhonghua Nei Ke Za Zhi* 38, no. 5 (May 1999): 302–305.

23. Rees, W. D., et al. "Effect of Deglycyrrhizinated Liquorice on Gastric Mucosal Damage by Aspirin." *Scandinavian Journal of Gastroenterology* 14, no. 5 (1979): 605–607.

24. "Aloe Vera." National Center for Complementary and Integrative Health, last modified Apr. 2012, https://nccih.nih.gov/health/aloevera.

25. Asadi-Shahmirzadi, A., et al. "Benefit of Aloe Vera and *Matricaria recutita* Mixture in Rat Irritable Bowel Syndrome: Combination of Antioxidant and Spasmolytic Effects." *Chinese Journal of Integrative Medicine* (Dec. 21, 2012): doi: 10.1007/s11655-012-1027-9.

26. Ranade, A. N.; N. S. Ranpise; and C. Ramesh. "Exploring the Potential Gastro Retentive Dosage Form in Delivery of Ellagic Acid and Aloe Vera Gel Powder for Treatment of Gastric Ulcers." *Current Drug Delivery* 11, no. 2 (2014): 287–97.

27. Cellini, L., et al. "In Vitro Activity of Aloe Vera Inner Gel Against *Helicobacter pylori* Strains." *Letters in Applied Microbiology* 59, no. 1 (July 2014): 43–8, doi: 10.1111/lam.12241.

28. Belluzzi, A., et al. "Effects of New Fish Oil Derivative on Fatty Acid Phospholipid-Membrane Pattern in a Group of Crohn's Disease Patients." *Digestive Diseases and Sciences* 39, no. 12 (Dec. 1994): 2589–94.

29. Gil, A. "Polyunsaturated Fatty Acids and Inflammatory Diseases." *Biomedicine and Pharmacotherapy* 56, no. 8 (Oct. 2002): 388–96.

30. Geerling, B. J., et al. "Comprehensive Nutritional Status in Recently Diagnosed Patients with Inflammatory Bowel Disease Compared with Population Controls." *European Journal of Clinical Nutrition* 54, no. 6 (June 2000): 514–21.

31. Fleming, C. R., et al. "Zinc Nutrition in Crohn's Disease." *Digestive Diseases and Sciences* 26, no. 10 (Oct. 1981): 865–70.

32. Yoga poses and how to meditate are explained in Chapter 8, but I wanted you to have a quick preview of what your morning would look like here.

33. I encourage all my patients to get their vitamins and minerals from a variety of vegetables in the diet, but if you feel that your diet is not varied enough in terms of the vegetables you eat (that is, you are deficient in the phytonutrient spectrum because you do not introduce enough variety into your diet), then you should take a daily B complex vitamin/multi-mineral formula to make up for any deficiencies in your diet.

34. Soak raw nuts in a 2:1 water-to-nut ratio for eight to twelve hours. Then rinse thoroughly and drain. Soaking and rinsing remove antinutrients, and sprouting (which takes longer, but is mostly used for seeds, not nuts) activates nutrients, neutralizes enzyme inhibitors that make nuts difficult to digest, and promotes the production of vital digestive enzymes.

35. Coconut oil by itself is a great way to balance blood sugar, prevent hypoglycemia between meals, satisfy hunger cravings, and feed the brain with medium-chain triglycerides, which provide excellent energy for attention and concentration.

36. An ayurvedic combination of three sour, astringent fruits (amalaki, bibhitaki, and haritaki) that has been used in India to support digestion, assimilation, and regularity. You will find that the capsule strengths vary. It is best to choose an organic supplement and start with a lower dose.

37. Ibid., note 33.

Chapter 4: Tips for Success: Creating a Happy Gut

1. Bonithon-Kopp, C., et al. "Calcium and Fibre Supplementation in Prevention of Colorectal Adenoma Recurrence: A Randomised Intervention Trial." *Lancet* 356, no. 9238 (Oct. 2000): 1300–306.

Part III: Reintroduction Phase and Further Testing
Chapter 5: Reintroduction and Your Gut C.A.R.E. Plan for Life

1. Corn is found in many gluten alternatives; however, be aware that corn metabolizes into sugar, which can trigger an insulin response, leading to weight gain and belly-fat accumulation. Just because it's gluten-free does not mean it's weight neutral. Introduce corn in moderation. Do not make it a staple in your diet.

2. Remember to use proper soaking techniques to reduce the phytate content of legumes.

Chapter 6: Further Testing for Gut-Related Ailments

1. I often find that patients seen by other doctors only have a TSH (thyroid stimulating hormone) level checked. TSH is produced by the pituitary to stimulate the thyroid to produce thyroid hormone. If thyroid hormone levels are low, the pituitary will secrete more TSH into the circulation to push the thyroid harder. The more affected your thyroid is, the higher your TSH levels will be. However, if you have borderline thyroid function, your TSH may look normal, while your T4 and free T3 (the unbound and most active form) levels may be abnormal. Or you may test positive for thyroid antibodies even though all values are normal and you are *not* exhibiting symptoms of thyroid malfunction yet. If you have normal thyroid function with elevated thyroid antibodies, you need to pull all inflammatory foods from your diet, including soy, dairy, and gluten. It's as simple as that. I have seen patients with autoimmune hyperthyroidism reverse their condition simply through these dietary measures without requiring medication to treat it.

2. See http://www.breakingtheviciouscycle.info/p/beginners-guide for more information about the Specific Carbohydrate Diet.

3. Halpern, G. M., and J. R. Scott. "Non-IgE Antibody Mediated Mechanisms in Food Allergy." *Annals of Allergy* 58, no. 1 (Jan. 1987): 14–27.

4. Atkinson, W., et al. "Food Elimination Based on IgG Antibodies in Irritable Bowel Syndrome: A Randomised Controlled Trial." *Gut* 53, no. 10 (Oct. 2004): 1459–64.

5. Lee, S. K., and P. H. Green. "Celiac Sprue (the Great Modern-Day Imposter)." *Current Opinion in Rheumatology* 18, no. 1 (Jan. 2006): 101–107.

6. Catassi, C., and A. Fasano. "Celiac Disease Diagnosis: Simple Rules Are Better Than Complicated Algorithms." *American Journal of Medicine* 123, no. 8 (Aug. 2010): 691–3.

7. Lin, H. C. "Small Intestinal Bacterial Overgrowth: A Framework for Understanding Irritable Bowel Syndrome." *JAMA* 192, no. 7 (Aug. 18, 2004): 852–8.

8. Quigley, E., and R. Quera. "Small Intestinal Bacterial Overgrowth: Roles of Antibiotics, Prebiotics, and Probiotics." *Gastroenterology* 130, no. 2, S1 (Feb. 2006): S78–90, doi:10.1053/j.gastro.2005.11.046.

9. Bouhnik, Y., et al. "Bacterial Populations Contaminating the Upper Gut in Patients with Small Intestinal Bacterial Overgrowth Syndrome." *American Journal of Gastroenterology* 94, no. 5 (May 1999): 1327–31.

10. Bures, J., et al. "Small Intestinal Bacterial Overgrowth Syndrome." *World Journal of Gastroenterology* 16, no. 24 (June 28, 2010): 2978–90.

11. Chang, C. S., et al. "Increased Accuracy of the Carbon-14 D-Xylose Breath Test in Detecting Small-Intestinal Bacterial Overgrowth by Correction with the Gastric Emptying Rate." *European Journal of Nuclear Medicine* 22, no. 10 (Oct. 1995): 1118–22.

Part IV: A Happy Gut, Happy Life
Chapter 7: The Emotional Gut: The Mind-Gut Connection

1. Banks, W. A., S. A. Farr, and J. E. Morley. "Entry of Blood-Borne Cytokines into the Central Nervous System: Effects on Cognitive Processes." *Neuroimmunomodulation* 10, no. 6 (2002–2003): 319–27.

2. Rivier, C. "Effect of Peripheral and Central Cytokines on the Hypothalamic-Pituitary-Adrenal Axis of the Rat." *Annals of the New York Academy of Sciences* 697 (Oct. 1993): 97–105.

3. Parracho, H. M., et al. "Differences Between the Gut Microflora of Children with Autistic Spectrum Disorders and That of Healthy Children." *Journal of Medical Microbiology* 54, no. 10 (Oct. 2005): 987–91.

Chapter 8: The Physical Gut: The Body-Gut Connection

1. Clarke, S. F., et al. "Exercise and Associated Dietary Extremes Impact on Gut Microbial Diversity." *Gut* 62, no. 12 (Dec. 2014): 1913–20, doi: 10.1136/gutjnl-2013-306541.

2. Having your own yoga mat is also more hygienic, since you are not sharing the same mat used by countless other people, which can spread viruses, fungi (yeast), and bacteria.

3. Caution: Never perform breath work on a full stomach. Wait at least three hours after eating a meal or perform it on an empty stomach.

4. A mudra is a symbolic gesture or seal.

Part V: Fun in the Kitchen
Chapter 9: Happy Gut Recipes

1. Matcha is made from stone-ground green tea leaves. By using the whole leaf, it provides a powerful arsenal of vitamins, minerals, and antioxidants unmatched by regular green tea. It is a cancer fighter and fat burner.

2. Giblets stored in a plastic bag and stuffed inside the chicken cavity pose a health risk if the bag melts during cooking. Giblets may also be sautéed, broiled, or simmered (for a homemade chicken stock), but they should be prepared outside of the chicken to ensure they are cooked thoroughly. After cooking to an internal temperature of 165°F, giblets are ready and should be firm in texture. If you are saving giblets for later, they should be refrigerated or frozen immediately after removal.

INDEX

deep listening, 194
dehydration, 131
depression, 6, 41, 92, 189, 195–96, 199
desserts, 139–40
    recipes, 310–12
DGL (deglycyrrhizinated licorice), 104–5, *151,*
    152, 336, 340, 342
DHA (docosahexaenoic acid), 106–7
diabetes, 41, 44, 51, 70, 87, 145, 158
Diagnos-Techs Clinical and Research Labora-
    tory, 347–48
diagnostic tests, xi, 143–46
    based on symptoms and conditions, *147–52*
    celiac disease, 159–60
    dairy sensitivity, 161–62
    dysbiosis, 167–71
    food allergies, *147,* 154–55
    food sensitivities, 156
    H. pylori infection, 180–81
    lactose intolerance, 161
    leaky gut syndrome, *151,* 157
    pancreatic enzyme insufficiency, 185
    SIBO, 173–74
    specialty laboratories for Functional Testing,
        resources, 346–51
    ten most common, 144–46
    yeast overgrowth or candidiasis, 112, *152,*
        175–76
diarrhea, 25, 171
    common OTC medicinal culprits, 359
    dysbiosis and, 167
    FODMAP intolerance and, 164
    gluten and, 47, 157
    lactose intolerance and, 56, 161
    SIBO and, 172
    sleep and, 127
    tests and therapies, *148*
diet. *See also* Happy Gut Diet
    author's story, 2–4
    Gabriella's story, 30
    Julie's story, 1–2
    popular and fad, 25–26
    Standard American (SAD), 15, 61, 197
diet sodas, 44, *45*
digestion
    chewing your food, 125
    main enzymes, 90–91
    overview of, 12–15
    primary organs of, 13
Digestion GB, 340
digestive enzyme deficiencies, 183–84, 200
    causes of, 183
    diagnosing, 183
    symptoms of, 183, 184
Digestive Enzymes Ultra, 340

digestive enzyme supplements, 92–93, 130, *150,*
    151, 152, 201, 334, 335, 337, 340, 341
dinner
    beef and lamb entrées, 296–99
    chicken entrées, 289–95
    daily protocol, 112–13
    seafood entrées, 283–88
    vegetarian entrées and sides, 300–309
dishwashing soap, 88
distilled water, 85
Doctor's Data, 348
documentaries, recommended, 355–56
dopamine, 44
Downward Facing Dog Pose, *223,* 223–24, 232, *232*
drinking water, 84–86
    for acid reflux, 130
    for constipation, 132
    with fiber intake, 101
    recommendations for improving, 84–85
    while eating, 125
drug metabolites, in drinking water, 84–85
Dunwoody Labs, 348
D-xylose breath tests, 173–74
dysbiosis, 22, *22,* 165–71. *See also* SIBO
    brain health and, 192, 196–97
    causes of, 166
    diagnosing, 167–71
    symptoms of, 167

eating alone, 124
eating principles, 123–26
eczema
    corn sensitivity and, 65–66
    DGL for, 105
    dysbiosis and, 167
    food sensitivities and, 155
    tests and therapies, *147*
eggs, 60–61, 64
    in Reintroduction Phase, 137–38, *139*
Eight-Point Pose, 231, *231*
electrolyzed oxidized (EO) water, 85
electrolyzed reduced (ER) water, 85
Elimination Phase. *See* Phase I of Happy Gut
    Diet
ELISA (enzyme-linked immunosorbent assay),
    156, 170, 171
ELISA/ACT Biotechnologies, 349
emotional eating, 209
emotional gut. *See* mind-gut connection
endoscopic biopsy, 181
energy levels, 31, 32
    sugar and, 41, 43
Enhance portion of Gut C.A.R.E. Program, 32,
    77, 102–8
    aloe vera, 105–6

InterFase Plus, 337
intestinal lining, repairing, regenerating, and
    healing. *See* Enhance portion of Gut
    C.A.R.E. Program
Ipecac 30C, 335
iron profile with ferritin tests, 144
irritable bowel syndrome (IBS), 3, 25, 203
    aloe vera for, 106
    antibiotics and dysbiosis, 22
    author's story, 3–4
    carrageenan and, 57
    Julie's story, 1–2, 143
    lactose intolerance and, 160, 161
    low-FODMAP diet for, 162, 163
    serotonin and, 195
    SIBO and, 171
    tests and therapies, *148, 150–51*

journals
    Pre-Program Four-Day Food/Symptom,
        313–14
    Twenty-Eight-Day Happy Gut Diet Food/
        Symptom, 79, 315–26

kale, 248, 282
Katrovas, Krista, 206
Kava Kava Root, 336
kefirs, 96, 138
    recipe, 259
kitchen makeover, 86–88
Klaire Labs, 336–37

laboratory tests. *See* diagnostic tests
lactase, 56
Lactobacillus, 95, 96–97, 102
lactoferrin, 170
lactose, 56, 162, 163
lactose intolerance, 56, 160–61
    cultured foods, 95–96
    vs. dairy sensitivity, 160
    diagnosing, 161
    testing protocols, 161
lamb
    recipe, 298
    resources, 351–52
leaky gut (leaky gut syndrome), 24–25, 156–57,
    192
    author's story, 3–4
    blood brain barrier and, 192, 196, 198–200
    common OTC medicinal culprits, 360
    conditions leading to, 24
    diagnosis, *151,* 157
    dysbiosis and, 22, *22*
    food sensitivities and, 25–26
    healthy gut vs., *23*
    lectins and, 52

probiotics and, 95
symptoms of, 25, 156
tests and therapies, *151,* 157
lectins, 51–53
    in corn, 65
    in legumes, 67
    in nightshades, 69
    in peanuts, 68
legumes, 51, 67–68, 100
    making less gassy, 68
    in Reintroduction Phase, 138, *139*
lemon juice, for smoothies, 248
leptin resistance, 52, 65
Levine, Stephen, 334
L-glutamine, 104, 105, 106, *148, 151,* 340, 342, 343
licorice root, 104–5
lifestyle and a happy gut, 127–28
lipases, 13, 90
linolenic acid, 68
listening to your gut, 194
liver, 13, 43, 91
liver cancer, 28
Liver-G.I. Detox, 340
Liver Health, 336
locally-grown foods, 83
long, deep breath, 238–39
loose stools. *See also* diarrhea
    tests and therapies, *148*
low stomach acid (hypochlorhydria), 91–92,
    181–83
    causes of, 91
    problems associated with, 91–92
    self-test for, 182–83
    symptoms of, 182
lunch, daily protocol, 111
Lunge Pose, 230, *230,* 233, *233*

magnesium citrate, 114, 132, *149*
magnesium citrate, 337
magnesium glycinate, *150, 151*
MALT (mucosa-associated lymphoid tissue),
    28, 180
maltitol, 164
mammalian nature, 206–7, 208–9
mannitol, 164
massage therapies, 203, 204
matcha, 247, 373*n*
meal plans, 117–21, 129
medication-induced GI distress, 185
medication side effects, 359–60
MediClear Plus, 341
meditation
    beginning yoga session with, 214, 215
    daily protocol, 110, 114, 202, 215
    the gut and, 194, 201–2
    nervous system and, 211